# SOCIAL WORK COMPETENCES

# New Directions in Social Work

## Series Editor: Antony A. Vass

Recent changes in the training requirements for social workers and allied professionals have prompted the need for a set of textbooks to address issues of knowledge, skills and practice as well as contemporary social debates. *New Directions in Social Work* is designed to cater for students' academic and professional needs, and, in the context of new course guidelines, will address specific areas of practice such as working with offenders; social problems and social policy; children and young people; families; people with specific needs; and working within the community.

# SOCIAL WORK COMPETENCES

Core Knowledge, Values and Skills

*edited by*
Antony A. Vass

SAGE Publications
London • Thousand Oaks • New Delhi

First published 1996
Reprinted 1997

 SAGE Publications Ltd
6  Bonhill Street
London EC2A 4PU

SAGE Publications Inc
2455 Teller Road
Thousand Oaks, California 91320

SAGE Publications India Pvt Ltd
32, M-Block Market
Greater Kailash – I
New Delhi 110 048

**British Library Cataloguing in Publication Data**

A catalogue record for this book is
available from the British Library.

ISBN 0 8039 7799 9
ISBN 0 8039 7800 6 (pbk)

**Library of Congress catalog record available**

Typeset by Mayhew Typesetting, Rhayader, Powys
Printed in Great Britain by Biddles Ltd, Guildford and King's Lynn

# Contents

# For Dimitris Layios

*Like a wreath around your face*
*The colour purple left a trace*
*Of life and death playing a game*
*Of love and hate*
*You tasted death, but chose life*
*You drunk the immortals' wine*
*To stay for ever alive and divine*

('Mauve', Andonis)

# Acknowledgements

The authors and publishers wish to thank the Department of Health for permission to reproduce copyright material from H. Giller (1993) *Children in Need* (Table, 'Levels of Prevention', p. 13) for Chapter 4 in this book. Our special thanks go to Jim Brown, Child Care Group, the Social Services Inspectorate, Department of Health, for his friendly and very supportive response to our request; and to the author, Dr Henri Giller, for permitting us to use aspects of his work. At the same time we would like to extend our appreciation to Dr Pauline Hardiker from whom Dr Henri Giller obtained the information on primary, secondary and tertiary levels of prevention.

We would also like to thank the London Borough of Greenwich for permitting, under the Council's 'Discipline and Efficiency Rules and Procedures', Beverley Morgan to contribute Chapter 5 in this book. We appreciate that the chapter is the author's own work and the Council accepts no responsibility for the author's opinion or conclusion.

Jenny Bonfield and Kate Jarvis in the School of Social Work and Health Sciences deserve lots of appreciation for their help in typing Chapter 5 and transferring material on to Wordperfect for editorial work. They are marvellous!

Finally, we are grateful to Rosemary Campbell, Jane Evans, Gillian Stern, Karen Phillips and Beth Humphries at Sage for their support and advice.

# Notes on Contributors

**Helen Cosis Brown** is Principal Lecturer at Middlesex University where she is the Programme Leader for the Master's in Social Work, Postgraduate Diploma in Social Work and the Diploma in Social Work courses. She was for nine years a social worker and team leader in an Inner London social services department. Her publications and research interests are in the area of sexuality and social work; working with lesbian and gay men in social work; and fostering and adoption.

**Jane Dutton** is Senior Lecturer in Social Work at Middlesex University and a staff member of the Institute of Family Therapy. Previously she worked for many years as a social worker and manager in local authority settings. Currently she teaches social work knowledge and skills, anti-discriminatory practice, family and group work, and work with children, young people and families. Her research interests are in the development of systemic thinking in child protection work, and in organisations. She has published in these areas (under the names of Conn and Dutton Conn), particularly focusing on gender and power differences.

**Ravi Kohli** is Senior Lecturer in Social Work at Middlesex University. His main teaching responsibilities and research interests focus on social work with children and families, within the framework of the Children Act 1989. Previously, he was, for a number of years, a generic social worker and a senior practitioner in children and families social work in London.

**Beverley Morgan** is Senior Care Manager, working with physically disabled and older people, in a London borough. Previously, she worked as a generic social worker, and with learning disabled and older people in residential and community-based projects for a number of years.

**Jennifer Pearce** is Principal Lecturer in Social Work at Middlesex University. She is the Programme Leader for the BA Social Science (DipSW) degree. Her teaching interests are in the delivery of anti-oppressive practice within social work and youth justice. Her research and publications address issues for young women within the youth justice system. She is currently involved in a research project concerned with urban safety and gender perspectives in crime prevention within an East London borough.

**Antony A. Vass** is Professor of Social and Penal Studies and Head of School of Social Work and Health Sciences at Middlesex University. He is professionally qualified in social work (probation studies) and has worked in various fields of social work as research worker, community worker, probationer psychologist and probation officer. He has published numerous articles in academic and professional journals, is the author of five books including *Alternatives to Prison* (Sage, 1990), and is editor (with Tim May) of *Working with Offenders: Issues, Contexts and Outcomes* (Sage, 1996). He is also co-writing a forthcoming book (with Geoffrey Pearson) on *Social Problems and Social Policy* (Sage, forthcoming).

# Introduction: The Quest for Quality

Social work and probation practice have always been in the news. Normally, their appearance in the media signals bad news. This bad news has been amplified by the numerous childcare inquiries which time and again have found social work knowledge and practice to be deficient and lacking in competence. In particular, social workers' repeatedly exposed (albeit in some instances inflated) failure to follow legal requirements, required standards, agency guidelines and procedural rules; their limited and dated knowledge of the law; and their lack of appropriate accountability brought disrepute, diminished confidence and demoralisation to a battered profession. At the same time such professional failures caused a public outcry and calls on the government to curtail the powers of social workers or to demand that they learn to be efficient and competent first before they are allowed to practise. Questions about social workers' training and the quality of that training began to be asked.

Social work and probation are, therefore, subject to considerable upheaval. On the one hand, there is pressure on the Central Council for Education and Training in Social Work (CCETSW) from central government to improve standards in social work and to ensure that such standards deliver value for money. In turn, CCETSW comes up with ideas, policies and requirements which are directed at programme providers (education and training establishments). These policies force programme providers to constantly return to the drawing board for revisions upon revisions of those rules. Social work in the United Kingdom is standing at the crossroads: there is a distinct unease that it will emerge out of this upheaval either as a stronger profession or, as some fear, a weaker and ineffective minor anomaly in the social and political structure of contemporary Britain.

Added to those concerns is the Home Office's expressed intention to alter probation officer recruitment and qualifying training by opening up recruitment to almost anyone who is prepared to consider working in the probation service and removing probation training from the higher education sector (Dews and Watts, 1994; Home Office, 1995a, 1995b). Although this is not an entirely foregone conclusion the very fact that it has re-established the old rifts between the role of the Home Office, CCETSW, social work, and higher education in the training of probation officers (for a critical discussion see Nellis, 1996) demonstrates that social work in this country is still going through significant stages of development and has not as yet reached, or been allowed to reach, a period of consolidation to establish itself as a full-blown, credible and reliable profession characterised by concreteness and distinctive purpose, structure, knowledge, values and skills.

This recognition of the lack of distinctive core knowledge, values and skills which social workers and probation officers could claim as their particular property and the means to deliver competent practice, prompted CCETSW to call for changes in the way in which social workers and probation officers are trained. Since 1989 CCETSW has pursued a crusade to introduce the amendments deemed necessary for raising standards and establishing a clear and credible purpose, a knowledge, value and skill base for all social workers including probation officers.

As a result, CCETSW introduced and approved a new qualification, the Diploma in Social Work (DipSW) as the professional qualification for social workers and probation officers in April 1989 and issued the *Rules and Requirements for the Diploma in Social Work*, Paper 30, in September 1989. The new qualification replaced two former CCETSW qualifying awards, the Certificate of Qualification in Social Work (CQSW) and the Certificate in Social Services (CSS). It was intended that the new award would 'signify that a student has attained a national standard based on an agreed statement of the knowledge, skills and values needed for competent social work practice' (CCETSW, 1991:5). CCETSW appealed to universities and colleges to 'work collaboratively with social work agencies as DipSW programme providers' (CCETSW, 1991:6) and made this a requirement for all programmes seeking approval.

At the time of approval, CCETSW also broadened the application of the new DipSW by incorporating into its declared interests and intentions the objective of accommodating and assimilating into the DipSW the development of vocational and professional qualifications offered by the National Council for Vocational Qualifications (NCVQ) and by the Scottish Vocational Education Council (SCOTVEC) and CCETSW in Scotland. CCETSW (1991:6) argued thus:

> The new DipSW needs siting in the wider arena of training for national vocational and professional qualifications . . . CCETSW has developed with others (particularly the Care Sector Consortium) a progressive framework of education and training in social work and social care leading to qualifications. New vocational qualifications and a post

qualifying advanced award are being introduced. Together with the DipSW, they will provide a progressive system of education, training and qualifications for the personal social services [including probation].

The Social Work Education and Training (DipSW) Rules 1990 were approved by the Privy Council in November 1990 and amended in June 1991. Similarly, the new Requirements for Probation Training in the DipSW in England and Wales were approved by Privy Council in June 1990. A second edition of Paper 30, stating the new requirements, was issued in September 1991.

The primary purpose of the DipSW, and hence the purpose of social work education and training, was stated by CCETSW to be the preparation of students for 'employment as professionally qualified social workers and probation officers' (CCETSW, 1991:8). That meant that the purpose of education and training was to create a body of knowledge, values and skills which would lead to social workers practising in a competent manner. The expectations of students (that is to say, the statement of requirements) made this objective very explicit. CCETSW clarified that the statement of requirements referred to the competences expected and required of all newly qualified social workers 'in all settings (field, residential, day, domiciliary, community and health care) and sectors (statutory, including probation and education, voluntary and private)' (CCETSW, 1991:9). Students were required to achieve and demonstrate core knowledge, values and skills; competence in assessing, planning, intervening and evaluating outcomes; competence in working with individuals, families and groups 'over a sustained period in an area of particular practice within the relevant legal and organizational framework'; and competence in transferring knowledge and skills from one situation to another irrespective of case, need, problem or context.

Hardly three years later and before programmes had time to assimilate, accommodate and apply the new regulations, the effectiveness of the DipSW was questioned and new amendments were called for. In January 1994, following central government's expressed concerns about 'political correctness' and particularly Paper 30's emphasis on anti-oppressive and anti-racist practice, CCETSW embarked on a fresh review of the DipSW in partnership with the Care Sector Consortium (CSC), the Occupational Standards Council for Health and Social Care. The new-found partnership with CSC 'recognised the Government's national standards programme and the remit of the CSC to develop national occupational standards'. A joint CCETSW/CSC Steering Group was set up and a group of consultants, including the National Institute for Social Work, was employed to 'develop national occupational standards for social workers on which to base the revision of the Statement of Requirements for the DipSW' (CCETSW, 1995:1). The Joint Steering Group's remit was (CCETSW, 1995:1):

1. to achieve contemporary relevance for the qualification, in the context of changing needs, legislation and service delivery;
2. to establish more consistent standards at outcome than on the present DipSW;
3. to provide a sound professional base for a career in social work, firmly located in higher education;
4. to secure the DipSW in the continuum of qualifications; and
5. to promote flexible opportunities for access to the education, training and qualification.

On 23 February 1995, CCETSW Council approved the revised DipSW and produced the first working copy of the new DipSW rules and requirements (CCETSW, 1995). It curtailed references to anti-discriminatory and anti-racist practice and focused, instead, on an Equal Opportunities Statement limited to four paragraphs. It redefined the purpose, knowledge, values and skills of the profession and presented a set of competences and practice requirements which should be satisfied by all qualifying students. The new requirements were meant not only to improve standards but also to promote wider and more flexible routes to education and training toward the DipSW: at non-graduate, undergraduate, postgraduate, college- or university-based, employment-based, modular, distance learning and part-time programmes.

In declaring the relevance and professional status of the new DipSW, CCETSW (1995:3; emphasis in original) argued thus:

> The Diploma in social Work is *the* professional social work qualification for social workers and probation officers; for social workers in all settings (residential, field, day, domiciliary, health care and criminal justice) and sectors (statutory, including education, voluntary and private) and for probation officers. . . . The DipSW is a UK qualification . . . at higher education level. . . . The DipSW prepares students for employment as professionally qualified social workers and probation officers *and* lays the foundation for their continuing professional development. The knowledge, values and skills required for competent social work practice for the award of the DipSW are set out in full. . . . The main features of the qualification are . . . to prepare students for work . . . and to prepare them to anticipate and respond to future changes in need, policy and service delivery.

Whether the above claims are sustainable it is too early to know. However, statements about competent practice which incorporate core knowledge, values and skills applicable to every setting and sector of work are one thing. Identifying those core elements, discussing them, applying them and constantly upgrading or updating them to fit changes in 'need, policy and service delivery' is another. There is a serious gap between good intent and actual practice. Although there are many written statements on diverse issues in social work and about competences, there is none which brings together, in a critical, informative and practically helpful manner, the links between knowledge, values and skills and the emergence of competent practice. And this is where the present textbook comes in.

We strongly believe that this book is novel in its approach and content. It addresses CCETSW's intentions and concerns and those of many others – from students and educators to trainers and employers. How can students understand the purpose of their tasks? How can they learn to search for and absorb relevant knowledge? How can they be taught and understand the values of their profession, and how do those values guide their work? How can students be shown how to develop skills relevant to effective practice? How can they be made to appreciate and practise in a holistic way, that is to say, by developing abilities which allow them to integrate knowledge, values and skills in order to produce competent practice? Finally, how can they be made to know what competences are important, what their components are and how those competences can be recognised in the quest for efficiency and quality?

In this book we have tried to address those questions in a structured way. We offer a critical account and discussion of the core knowledge, values and skills required by social workers and probation officers for understanding their tasks and duties and delivering reliable and efficient service. We then link those three elements to a discussion about *particular* areas of work, or *pathways* (a term used in the new DipSW: CCETSW, 1995). We have concentrated attention on three pathways: social work with children and families; community care and social work with adults; and crime, probation and social work with offenders. Each area is covered in some detail and readers will be helped to understand as well as apply some of the core requirements expected in each of those areas for competent practice. Finally, we offer a practical tool in identifying as well as monitoring competences. Having integrated the knowledge, values and skills to produce a set of competences, we operationalise those competences by stating their main components and indicators for readers to use as heuristic devices against which their own understanding and practice of competences can be monitored, measured, amended, transcended or improved.

In order to achieve the above lofty goals (in an area such as social work, which is well renowned for its ambiguity), a team of experienced social work academics and practitioners with expertise in each area covered was assembled to contribute to the book. Helen Cosis Brown covers, in Chapter 1, 'The Knowledge Base of Social Work'. The chapter discusses the historical context of social work's use of knowledge and major weaknesses; the relevance of applied social sciences; anti-discriminatory practice; knowledge which is essential and helps practitioners plan appropriate intervention; and how knowledge is an essential part of developing competent practice. In Chapter 2 Jennifer Pearce addresses the importance and relevance of 'The Values of Social Work' and demonstrates how those core values are essential requirements for an efficient and reliable social work and probation practice. In Chapter 3 Jane Dutton and Ravi Kohli take up the issue of 'The Core Skills of Social Work', identifying the core skills which every social worker and probation officer should be able to use in order to achieve appropriate outcomes.

The three areas are then integrated for a discussion around three particular pathways. In Chapter 4, Ravi Kohli and Jane Dutton cover major areas relevant to 'Social Work with Children and Families' and provide useful pointers for good practice. Chapter 5 follows a similar theme but in this instance with reference to 'Community Care and Social Work with Adults'. Here Beverley Morgan provides an historical account of discrimination against 'adults'; the emergence of community care; the effects of inefficient and sometimes incompatible knowledge, values and skills; care management as a needs-led process for assessment and planning; service user involvement; the disability movement's view of community care; and the knowledge, values and skills required for competent performance in this area of work. Antony Vass, in Chapter 6, offers a detailed discussion of the knowledge, values and skills required by probation officers and those working with offenders for effective and efficient practice. The chapter, 'Crime, Probation and Social Work with Offenders', also covers the relevance of criminology and penal policy, theories of crime and deviance, the organisational context of the criminal justice system, sentencing and national standards, child protection and the effectiveness of intervention.

Finally, in Chapter 7 Antony Vass brings the first part of the book – the knowledge, values and skills – and the second part – the three pathways – together to offer an integrative model of work that combines the various types of core knowledge, values and skills to produce a set of required competences. These competences are then operationalised; in other words they are defined in terms of their major components and indicators to guide the reader towards an understanding of what competences mean and what they may imply in practice. The chapter concludes by suggesting that it is not the tasks that social workers and probation officers do that matters but how they carry out those tasks and to what effect.

In conclusion, we believe that this book will prove useful and helpful to all social work and probation students, their teachers and practitioners (and any other individual or agency, including perhaps CCETSW and the Home Office) in their studies, practice and policies. It may also assist understanding of social work and the probation service's purpose, and how competent practice can be achieved and attained.

Irrespective of the state or outcome of current debates about social work and probation practice, current and future students will find this book both relevant and useful to their professional needs.

### References

CCETSW (1991) *DipSW: Rules and Requirements for the Diploma in Social Work* (Paper 30), 2nd edn. London: Central Council for Education and Training in Social Work.

CCETSW (1995) *DipSW: Rules and Requirements for the Diploma in Social Work* (Paper 30), revised edn. London: Central Council for Education and Training in Social Work.

Dews, V. and Watts, J. (1994) *Review of Probation Officer Recruitment and Qualifying Training*. London: Home Office.

Home Office (1995a) *Review of Probation Officer Recruitment and Qualifying Training. Discussion Paper*. London: Home Office (mimeo).

Home Office (1995b) *Review of Probation Officer Recruitment and Qualifying Training. Decision Paper by the Home Office*. London: Home Office (mimeo).

Nellis, M. (1996) 'Probation training: the links with social work', in T. May and A.A. Vass (eds), *Working with Offenders: Issues, Contexts and Outcomes*. London: Sage. pp. 7–30.

# 1

# The Knowledge Base of Social Work

The relationship between social work practice and knowledge has always been ambivalent, sometimes even dismissive. The social work profession emphasises the need to link theory and practice, making this ability a requirement for qualification. It has been argued that the 'insistence that theory and practice are complementary aspects of the same thing is part of a verbal rather than a real tradition in social work' (Sheldon, 1978:1). Other research shows that few social workers inform their work with theory, being more likely to rely on their own experience or advice from colleagues (Carew, 1979). Sheldon's work uncovered two distinct subcultures within social work, a theoretical one and a practice one. Findings of work undertaken by the theoretical subculture are either not believed, by the practice subculture, or 'are seen as the products of a process which has little direct relevance to the practice situation' (Sheldon, 1978:2). Although nearly two decades have passed since Sheldon and Carew were writing in this area their conclusions may still be true.

The use of knowledge is, not surprisingly, subjective. We are much more likely to seek out knowledge to retrospectively justify our practice and decision-making, rather than acquiring knowledge, beforehand, to inform our intervention. Social workers sometimes use selective knowledge to reinforce decisions that have been reached on the basis of their belief system or value base (Brown, 1992a). This tendency has led to discriminatory practice. The knowledge that is used by practitioners may in itself be problematic. Research findings based on small samples with methodologically questionable approaches have occasionally established themselves as universal truths in social work, with little foundation. Parton and others have helpfully questioned some of these 'truths' within the area of child protection (Parton, 1985; Violence against Children Study Group, 1990). It is now generally accepted, as a result of the growing anti-discriminatory practice literature, that knowledge informing practice has often been relevant only to particular groups in society and the indiscriminate use of such knowledge has contributed to, rather than alleviated, clients' and service users' oppression (Brown, 1991; Bryan, 1992; Channer and Parton, 1990; Thompson, 1993).

Discussions about the knowledge base of social work may therefore realistically be about what is considered relevant to practitioners, rather than what actually does inform their practice. However, there has been nothing, within the profession, like the fear generated over the last decade by the numerous childcare inquiries (Department of Health, 1991b; Heder et al., 1993), to sharpen thinking as to why knowledge is relevant to social work practice. The findings of the Jasmine Beckford inquiry (London Borough of Brent, 1985) revealed practitioners to be lacking in the six areas that Payne identifies as showing how theory has something to offer practice: models; approaches to or perspectives on; explanations; prescriptions; accountability and justifications (Payne, 1991:52). In addition, the panel of inquiry looking into the death of Tyra Henry (London Borough of Lambeth, 1987) identified specific gaps in the knowledge base informing the practice of those involved. The panel felt there had been insufficient consideration of the impact of loss on the individuals concerned and as a result the models, approaches, explanations and prescriptions had all been tragically flawed. What the childcare inquiries told both the profession and the public was that ill-informed practice at best leads to incompetence and at worst to loss of life.

There are many factors which contributed to the overhaul of social work education and training in Britain in the late 1980s, culminating in the new social work qualification, the Diploma in Social Work (CCETSW, 1989, 1991). A major factor was the loss of public confidence in social work's credibility, resulting from the childcare inquiries. Social work as a profession required more clarity in its expectations for qualifying social workers in relation to knowledge. It needed to be clear about what knowledge was useful in relation to its roles, responsibilities and tasks, as set out under the three major pieces of legislation relevant to these: the Children Act 1989, the Criminal Justice Act 1991 and the National Health Service and Community Care Act 1990. This chapter attempts to bring together under three headings, relating to these pieces of legislation, areas of knowledge and theory that need to be part of a social worker's 'tool kit' for competent practice.

Social workers, approaching any piece of work, have to ask themselves, and be able to answer, three simple questions: what am I going to do?, why am I going to do it? and how will it be accomplished? To be able to answer these questions, the social worker needs to be familiar with the knowledge base of social work. Numerous models have been developed to facilitate both an organisation and an understanding of social work knowledge (Barker and Hardiker, 1981; Coulshed, 1991; Hanvey and Philpot, 1994; Howe,

1987; Payne, 1991). The different methods of organisation and understanding offered suit the needs of some and not of others. What is striking about the social work literature in this area are two things: first that there is often a confusing interchangeable use of the terms 'theory', 'knowledge' and 'methods'; and secondly that texts about social work theory and knowledge are primarily about methods and models of social work intervention.

This chapter is organised under three headings that made sense to the author of this chapter when she worked as a team leader in a generic social services team, when trying to help the team answer the what, why and how questions; and when preparing for or reflecting on the team's intervention with clients and service users. These three distinct areas are: knowledge that informs the practitioner about the client's experience and context; knowledge that helps the practitioner plan appropriate intervention; and knowledge that clarifies the practitioner's understanding of the legal, policy, procedural and organisational context in which their practice takes place. The section addressing knowledge that informs the practitioner about clients' experience and context will draw on three perspectives – sociological, psychological and anti-discriminatory values and practice. The second section, knowledge that helps the practitioner plan appropriate intervention, will review methods and models of social work intervention and the theories that inform them. The last section, knowledge that clarifies practitioners' understanding of the legal, policy, procedural and organisational context in which their practice takes place, will relate to the three major pieces of legislation concerning probation and offenders, adults in need of support services, and children and families. At the same time the discussion will consider legal processes with which practitioners need to be familiar in order to be competent.

By the very enormity of the knowledge base of social work this chapter should be seen as a series of signposts, indicating areas of significance to be explored further through other identified helpful texts. Many of these signposts relate to particular areas of practice that will be examined in the chapters which follow.

Before embarking on the main body of this chapter it would be helpful to place the whole question of social work's use of knowledge in its historical context. This will help to establish the connections between the three sections identified above.

## The historical context of social work's use of knowledge

The author of this chapter once heard social workers described by an eminent professor as 'raving eclectics'. She did not approve of eclecticism, and was not alone in seeing it as one of the fundamental weaknesses of the social work profession. Payne (1991) helpfully identifies a series of positives and negatives associated with eclecticism. This chapter reflects on one of the positive aspects he identifies. 'Clients', he says 'should be able to benefit from all available knowledge so theoretical perspectives should not be limited' (Payne, 1991:51). This needs to be the case, as social work covers the full range of human experience and circumstances. However, it does make thinking about the knowledge base feel both infinite and unmanageable. Little wonder that the expectation that they can master so much makes social workers fall back on their 'common sense'. It is as though they rationalise that they cannot know everything about all things human and 'common sense' comes to the rescue as a solution to their predicament. Indeed it seems like an instrumental adjustment – a conscious act of coping in the face of the unknown.

In reality things are not quite as chaotic as might be feared. The roles, responsibilities and tasks of social work are defined by legislation. So it becomes a matter for the profession of defining what knowledge is relevant to its practice within a particular social, historical and cultural context. Social work, being a socially constructed activity, needs to be part of and understood within an interactive and dynamic process of becoming. This is essential, both within the profession and between itself and service users, if social work is to define an appropriate knowledge base.

In Britain, since the 1930s, social work, in its efforts to develop into a profession, has sought out an appropriate and applicable body of knowledge to draw on that would increase its credibility (Payne, 1992; Pearson et al., 1988; Yelloly, 1980). In this search, during the 1940s and 1950s, it is not surprising that it turned to psychoanalytic ideas, as social work and psychoanalysis were both, at that time, concerned with developing theory and bettering practice in the areas of attachment and loss. But the image of a profession of female social workers – as of course they were, as indeed they still primarily are (Howe, 1986) – calmly reflecting on the analytic process with their clients is something of a myth. Social work by its very nature has always had a significant element of pragmatism, involving itself, as it has to, with the detail of people's day-to-day existence as well as their innermost feelings. Pearson et al. (1988:4) explain that the influence of psychoanalytic ideas in social work 'never even approached a psychoanalytic takeover; British social work was too firmly rooted in the Tawney tradition of democratic socialism for that to be a possibility'. However, psychoanalytic ideas, rather than psychoanalytic method, did influence social work and laid the foundations for the diagnostic and social casework which dominated approaches to social work intervention for at least two decades (Payne, 1992).

Psychodynamic ideas were largely abandoned in the 1960s. This was for a number of reasons, including the sometimes crude misuse and rigid application of these ideas. As a body of theory they did not easily translate into a social work method and it was difficult to prove their effectiveness. The psychodynamic approach was too individualistic in its assessments of clients' circumstances; its method of social casework was no longer cost-effective and the recipients of psychodynamic casework very often had no understanding of what was going on, or of the purpose of the social work intervention (Mayer and Timms, 1970).

Social workers' growing scepticism about the practical relevance of psychodynamic ideas to their work coincided with the growing credibility and apparent relevance of two separate disciplines: sociology and psychology. This happened at the same time as an increasing number of graduates and postgraduates entered social work (from the 1960s onwards), many of whom had studied these disciplines. During this period sociology and psychology were interested in pursuing positivistic scientific methods of understanding and research, which were both objective and measurable. This offered a very different perspective from the subjective nature of psychodynamic ideas. It was thought that these disciplines would be able to offer objective explanations of clients' lives and circumstances. During the same period there were a number of developing theories and methods of intervention based on conscious processes which were seen as directly relevant to social work practice. These included problem-solving and crisis intervention theory, task-centred work, systems theory and behavioural approaches, to name a few.

The social and political upheavals of the late 1960s had a profound impact on academic disciplines and social work knowledge and practice. Phenomenology was influential within psychology and sociology and as a result on social work theory. Marxism, interactionism, structuralism and construct theory had an impact on the development of radical social work ideas of the 1970s (Brake and Bailey, 1980; Langan and Lee, 1989; Statham, 1978). As with psychodynamic ideas, it would be difficult to measure the impact radical social work had on actual practice. However, it was to have an influence on the development of different perspectives and ideas within social work theory and practice. It raised the awareness of class as a fundamentally important concept within social work. By its omission of race and gender from its discourse (with some exceptions), it ironically made a contribution to the mushrooming of anti-discriminatory practice ideas in precisely those areas in the 1980s. It is noteworthy that in the 1990s we have feminist social work knowledge and practice (Hanmer and Statham, 1988; Dominelli and McLeod, 1989; Langan and Day, 1992), and anti-racist social work (Ahmad, 1990; Dominelli, 1988; Husband, 1991; Hutchinson-Reis, 1989) but no equivalent body in relation to class. In the late 1980s and the early 1990s class politics (presumably partly due to the rise of the New Right and the fall of socialist states) was no longer in vogue, but identity politics was.

The eclecticism referred to at the beginning of this section is a reflection of social work's flirtation with different developing ideas since the 1930s. Social work has reflected the changing social, cultural and historical context in which it has practised, and sought out applicable knowledge accordingly. Today we have a whole range of ideas and methods employed by different practitioners working within different contexts, including the re-evaluation and reclamation by some practitioners and agencies of psychodynamic ideas.

### Knowledge that informs the practitioner about the client's experience and context

Social work has drawn on a number of different areas, including anti-discriminatory practice, psychology and the social sciences. There are many overlapping ideas and themes between all three, particularly between sociology and anti-discriminatory practice. It may seem inaccurate to describe anti-discriminatory practice as a discrete body of knowledge, but over the last few years a significant literature has developed, which merits attention in its own right.

*Sociology, social problems and social policy*
These three areas are separate but interrelated. Sociological ideas and theories have helped to facilitate an understanding of social problems, which in turn has had some impact on the formulation of social policy (see for instance Downes and Rock, 1988; Pearson, 1975; Vass, 1984, 1986, 1990). It would seem that all three areas are relevant to social work. It has been argued that social work has been about the amelioration of social ills not about challenging or even questioning oppression that might contribute to them (Jordan and Parton, 1983). If this has been the case CCETSW, in the late 1980s, by placing structural issues at the core of social work education and training, was challenging how social work education had tradition-ally been delivered.

Burrell and Morgan developed a helpful framework of paradigms that facilitates an understanding of the relationships between different sociological debates: between radical humanists, radical structuralists, interpretivists and functionalists (Burrell and Morgan, 1979). Although there have been various comments about the limitations of this framework (Rojek, 1986; Stenson and Gould, 1986), it can make manageable, for social workers, different and often conflicting sociological traditions and debates. Howe (1987) develops these ideas to locate different social work theories within each paradigm. However we structure the study of ideas, they need to be located within their historical, social and cultural contexts, as their perceptions of individuals, families and communities are accompanied by sets of interrelated values. These ideas can be difficult to translate into relevant material for informing social work practice, but this has been accomplished (Rojek et al., 1988). Ideas drawn from sociology, social theory and political theory offer practitioners ways of understanding the society and institutions within which they practise and the individuals, families and groups with whom they work. One of the major ways sociology has contributed to social work has been by its contribution to an understanding of social problems, the centre of practitioners' daily routine. At the same time sociological knowledge has introduced a challenging critique of the state, its administrative machines (for instance bureaucracy), its penal institutions (e.g. courts, prisons and the police), inequalities in health, education and employment, and has also raised questions about the professions' (e.g. social work) caring and controlling aspects. Sociological ideas helped shift social work from a position of pathologising individuals, to seeking a broader understanding of the problems with which they were faced. An understanding of poverty, crime, mental illness, deviance, substance abuse, racism and violence has been facilitated by the input of sociological theories into social work's knowledge base. The development of ideas about anti-discriminatory practice started for a number of different reasons, but the contribution of sociology is indisputable.

In complex ways, which are neither linear nor causal, society's understanding of social problems, partly aided by sociological concepts and ideas, is eventually translated into social policy. For example Goffman's critical analysis of institutions (Goffman, 1961), albeit with its own ideological and methodological flaws, contributed, in ways that would be difficult to measure, to the increased pressure from all sides of the political spectrum for a move towards vulnerable individuals remaining in the community wherever possible. This pressure was eventually actualised in the Mental Health Act 1983 and the National Health Service and Community

Care Act 1990. Interrelated with the critique of 'total institutions' was a parallel sociological critique of prisons, as well as calls for new community penalties for the treatment of offenders (Vass, 1990), which culminated in the Criminal Justice Act 1991. Although it is easy to extol the influence of sociological knowledge and research on policy and practice at the cost of ignoring or neglecting sociopolitical and economic contingencies in the formation of social and penal policy (see for instance Scull, 1984), the relevance of such knowledge remains strong. Feminist analysis has acted as a catalyst in developing social policy initiatives that are more sympathetic to women and children (Maclean and Groves, 1991). The study of social policy has enabled practitioners to have an appreciation of the historical development of welfare provision, leading to a more complex understanding of the current contexts of social work and probation practice and provision.

Fundamental to social work is the practitioner's understanding of what clients may share in common and what may be beyond their individual power to change. Sociology makes a unique contribution to this. *In toto*, sociological perspectives and policy studies may not have an immediate practical value to the social worker but they manage, to use Vass's phrase, 'to galvanize social workers' consciousness about the society, the political and social context within which they work. Sociology may not offer social workers immediate practical tools, but it certainly makes them more informed and competent professionals' (Vass, 1987).

*Psychology*
Sociology offers the practitioner an understanding of social processes, society, systems and institutions, while psychology offers explanations of individuals' behaviour and relationships with others. As with sociology, there are numerous traditions and debates within psychology. Social work has often organised its use of psychological ideas within two separate frameworks: human growth and development or developmental psychology; and abnormal psychology or psychopathology. The first has drawn on psychoanalytic psychology, particularly ego-psychology, for example the work of Erikson (1965), and the British School of object relations (Winnicott, 1964). Social work's understanding of abnormal psychology has been more reliant on behavioural psychology and psychiatry (Clare, 1980).

This organisation of psychological ideas relevant to practitioners has helped to make a very broad area of study manageable. Social workers need a working understanding of human development to be able to make an informed assessment of their particular clients' circumstances. By the nature of their work practitioners have to be familiar with abnormal psychology, for they will be working, in some circumstances, with people who are mentally disordered, and also have to be able to identify someone who is in need of intervention in order to prevent emotional deterioration, and to differentiate normal human distress from the abnormal.

Social workers are not expected to be amateur psychologists or psychiatrists. They are expected, however, to be familiar enough with psychological ideas to draw on them to make informed assessments and then to plan effective intervention. Practitioners who act as approved social workers under the Mental Health Act 1983 receive an additional post-qualifying training before they undertake their duties.

Different branches of psychology have their own contributions to make. Behavioural psychology has offered models of understanding behaviour and models of change that have proved useful in a number of ways. For example, the management of anxiety; managing agoraphobia; working with parents of enuretic children and the management of problematic substance use. Social learning theory (Bandura, 1977) has contributed to aiding the independence of people with learning difficulties, using such techniques as chaining (Tsoi and Yule, 1982). Cognitive-developmental approaches (Piaget, 1952) have made an impact on the consideration of environmental factors necessary to children's development, proving important in work with children and families. Social psychology draws on both psychoanalytic psychology and behavioural psychology, while contributing its own unique perspectives on individuals within groups and organisations. Social psychological ideas have been relevant to social work in many ways, including the understanding of social work agencies and their processes (Nicholson and Bayne, 1990).

Like social work's relationship with sociology, practice benefits from the study of the different schools of thought within psychology in their applied and abstract forms. Psychology has a lot to offer the practitioner in relation to specific problems and life events. As well as giving a general understanding of human beings' behaviour and experience, it can contribute to social workers' effective intervention.

Psychology has been profoundly influential in the development of ideas around attachment, separation and loss (see for instance Bowlby, 1988; Kubler-Ross, 1973; Parkes, 1972; Robertson and Robertson, 1989; Worden, 1983). Work with which social workers engage usually involves some aspects of attachment, separation and loss. These areas of psychological thought have contributed to work with families; child protection; planning for children being cared for; assessment of adults in relation to community care; bereavement work, and through-care of prisoners.

Psychology and sociology have both proved to be essential, integral parts of the knowledge base of social work, enabling a complex understanding of clients' circumstances. Their offerings and approaches do not have to be mutually exclusive. They enable a thorough assessment and understanding of a presenting situation and help the practitioner to consider the most appropriate response. For social workers to be able to practise competently they also need to have an understanding of social research methods and methodology; this allows them to assess the relevance and usefulness of research to their practice as well as to be constructively critical of their own practice. However, knowledge and its use is never a neutral affair, divorced from its cultural, social and historical roots and specificity. Anti-discriminatory practice and theory have made an invaluable contribution to the necessary process of re-evaluating social work knowledge.

*Anti-discriminatory practice*
Social work has stood accused of being, either by design or by default, an oppressive institution (Oliver, 1991; Langan and Day 1992; Dominelli, 1988). Both the structures of social work provision, in their various guises, and social work practice itself have come under scrutiny. The components of competent practice, knowledge, values and skills have attracted very different amounts of attention from critics of social work's discriminatory practice. Values have often been the focal point for such discussions. There were, quite rightly, questions asked about how social workers' own beliefs, attitudes and values impacted in a detrimental fashion on their clients. Although Chapter 2 on social work values explores this in more depth, it is both relevant and necessary to cover the theme briefly from a different angle here.

Earlier in this chapter it was proposed that social workers, like many others, might seek out knowledge that sat comfortably with their personal values and preconceived ideas. The content of much social work practice makes objectivity a difficult thing. Ryburn argues that in assessments of prospective adoption and fostering applicants, striving for professional objectivity may be problematic if not impossible. It is more honest and helpful, therefore, to declare our subjectivity (Ryburn, 1991). It may indeed be in clients' and service users' interests for social workers to be aware of and declare their subjectivity, but clients also need to be reassured that the practitioner has taken cognisance of various perspectives on a given situation to enable them to undertake informed decision-making, for which they will be accountable. Social work's relationship with knowledge is problematic because of the complex interrelationships of knowledge, values and practice and the difficult interpretative processes at play, as well as the often diverse and conflicting interests which have to be defined and accommodated in any decision-making context.

Knowledge itself may be problematic. Knowledge is a product of a specific social, cultural and historical moment. It is not always fact, and it is not finite, but needs to be a dynamic, flexible entity if it is to be useful to social workers and their clients. Anti-discriminatory practice debates have been invaluable in contributing to the profession's own critical reappraisal of social work knowledge, by highlighting social work's occasional treatment of theory as if it were universal truth, often to the detriment of service users. Models developed to test out theories were sometimes applied as if they were the only reality, rather than being seen as possible ways of viewing human experience. Wilson was one of the first to explore this, examining social work's misuse and over-zealous, rigid application of psychodynamic ideas, particularly in relation to notions of femininity. Reviewing a 1950s social work text, she notes: 'The authors stress the importance of correct gender identifications and the neurosis and immaturity to which those who fail to become truly "masculine" or "feminine" are condemned' (Wilson, 1977:87).

Much has been written on the racist implications of the inappropriate application of some psychological theories, when their cultural specificity has been ignored. Phoenix, looking at theories, based on the experiences of white men and women, of how human beings become gendered, has reviewed the literature to examine its applicability to people of African-Caribbean descent (Phoenix, 1990). Difficulties arise when theories have not been reviewed in this way.

Another example of the need to re-examine social work knowledge has been the applicability of material about the ageing process and its relevance to lesbians and gay men (Berger, 1990; Brown, 1992). As Berger (1990:170) succinctly puts it, 'the professional literature on ageing gave one the impression that homosexuality did not exist among the elderly'. As a result of this, lesbians and gay men 'have been ignored by both gerontological researchers and by service providers'. Service provision and the quality of practice have a direct relationship with the knowledge base of social work. If the knowledge is flawed, or excludes whole communities, the outcome will in some cases be incompetent practice and inadequate or inappropriate service provision.

The work of the Women's Therapy Centre has been central to the reconsideration of mainstream psychology's contribution to making sense of women's experience (Eichenbaum and Orbach, 1983; Ernst and Maguire, 1987). The ideas that have been developed have in turn been influential in helping social workers re-evaluate their practice. Lawrence (1992:32) suggests that a 'deeper and more careful understanding of women's psychological development is essential if social workers are to find a more helpful response to women clients'.

For knowledge to have a meaningful relationship to practice, knowledge and practice need to be engaged in a mutually influential dialogue. When knowledge is considered that is relevant to a particular piece of work, it needs to be contextualised socially, culturally and historically. Sometimes this process has taken the form of fashionable whim, resulting in ill-informed rejection of important areas of knowledge. An example would be the rejecting cynicism with which much of Bowlby's work is viewed by some social work educators, students and practitioners. Bowlby's work conveys a view that reinforces the supremacy of the heterosexual family because he was reflecting the norms of the context in which he undertook his work. However, none of this negates the crucially important ideas he had about attachment and loss, which may be universally applicable with adaptations to meet the needs of different contexts (Bowlby, 1988).

There needs to be reflection on and a re-evaluation of the knowledge base of social work, as well as an encouraging climate for new writing and research by practitioners, academics, educators, trainers and students as well as service users, in the light of anti-discriminatory ideas and practice. Social work would be ill advised to 'throw the baby out with the bathwater'.

### Knowledge that helps the practitioner plan appropriate intervention

Practitioners need knowledge to assist them in formulating a complex assessment of a client's circumstances, experience and context. They should also be familiar with models of social work intervention and the processes involved in intervention. This is the area often referred to as social work knowledge, and it covers a confusing variety of theory, models and approaches, all subsumed under one heading. Some of these models and theories have been developed within social work, and some, like crisis intervention and systems theory, have been borrowed from other disciplines and adapted to fit different social work contexts. Within the social work literature there is often a lumping together of areas such as behavioural social work, group work, psychodynamic theory, assessment, review and evaluation, and systems theory. Clearly these are very different. Some, like systems theory, represent a whole body of theory which is then formulated into particular models of intervention, whereas group work can be seen as a method of social work intervention. Assessment can be understood as a process that is involved in social work intervention.

*Theories and models*
Currently social work represents a very different picture of knowledge and practice than that of the 1950s, when the dominant theory was the psychodynamic perspective. At the present time practitioners and clients have the benefit of a range of ideas that can inform the model of intervention they use. These theories and their resulting models do not have to be used exclusively, but can complement one another. They include: crisis theory, systems theory, psychodynamic theory and behavioural theory. From all of these there have developed corresponding models of intervention. Other models draw on various theoretical bases, for example task-centred work. Yet other approaches to social work have developed from political and social theories: these include anti-racist social work (Ahmed, 1994); feminist approaches (Hudson et al., 1994); radical and Marxist approaches (Payne, 1991); and participatory approaches to social work (Beresford and Croft, 1993). This list is by no means exhaustive. It is beyond the scope of this chapter to discuss the theories or elaborate on the models involved. There are excellent, well-referenced texts that offer helpful summaries for both practitioners and students (see for example Coulshed, 1991; Howe, 1987; Hanvey and Philpot, 1994; Lishman, 1991; Payne, 1991; Rojek et al., 1988).

As said earlier, the disciplines of psychology and sociology have a particular relevance to social work knowledge. This is nowhere more apparent than in social work theory and models. There is a very clear overlap between social work and psychology and sociology, to such an extent that they are often inseparable. Some social work models are developed from theories that have their basis in psychology. Crisis intervention is a case in point. O'Hagan's (1986) model of crisis intervention, which is probably the most applicable to social services and probation settings, draws on a number of theories and models, including systems theory and task-centred models. It has its roots firmly planted in the classical crisis theory and crisis intervention theory literature that developed within psychology and psychiatry in the 1960s (Parad, 1965), which in turn drew on psychological work developed in the 1940s (Lindermann, 1944). Social work theories and their resulting models have evolved over time and have responded to the changing contexts in which social work has been practised.

Theories and models are never separate from social, political and ideological meaning. Systems theory is an example of the complex interrelationship of ideology, theory and the resulting model of intervention. It shares many ideas with structural functionalism as well as with biology. Hall and Fagen describe a system as 'a set of objects together with relationships between the objects and between their attributes' (1956:18). Systems theory offers the social worker a perspective which encompasses both individuals and their social environment (Pincus and Minahan, 1973; Specht and Vickery, 1977). However, it is a theory and a model of intervention which, it has been argued, is concerned with helping (or destabilising) systems, whether they be families, teams or organisations, to function effectively and smoothly. It does not necessarily question whether or not the system itself is in the interests of all its component parts. Furthermore, the concept of 'system' can also be problematic, as it may denote a set of organised social relationships (where there may be few or none) and its scope is almost limitless. For example in terms of translating the model into action, it will be an infinite task constantly to define every possible 'system' in mapping out the relations and connections between contexts and participants. Feminists, developing a critical analysis of the family – arguing that the family, as a system, was flawed because of how it had developed under patriarchal capitalism and that as an institution it served the interests of men and capital and acted against the interests of women (Barrett and McIntosh, 1982) – have often been critical of systems theory and of how it has sometimes been enacted within systemic family therapy. Systems theory in its application to working with families, when it does not address the different members' differential access to power, is seen by some as fundamentally flawed and potentially oppressive to women and children. This debate has centred particularly on the use of systems theory in dealing with child sexual abuse (MacLeod and Saraga, 1987). More seriously, Pilalis and Anderton's criticism that 'family systemic therapy's weakness is in its failure to address the links between the family system and the social structure' (Pilalis and Anderton, 1986:104) limits opportunities to incorporate ideas from socialist feminism in family therapy, which would enable a systems approach to benefit all members of a family. There have been important contributions to systems theory which have tried to incorporate a social contextualisation (see Perelberg and Miller, 1990; Burck and Speed, 1995) into practice.

Social work's knowledge base, in relation to theories and methods, is evolving and changing over time, in response to criticism and new contributions. It is essential that practitioners maintain a flexible and critical approach. They must ensure that theories and models are helpful and do not become a set of 'blinkers' which create rigid and distorted impressions of social life's complexities.

*Methods of social work intervention*

Methods of intervention, and processes involved in social work intervention, are intimately connected. For example, assessment is a necessary stage in defining what method of intervention would be most effective. If an assessment is made of a carer who is experiencing isolation, consideration needs to be given as to whether an individual approach would be most beneficial or whether the carer would benefit from a group work approach, by being a member of a carers' support group.

Methods of intervention would include individual work, individual counselling, family work, group work and community work. Here these are described as methods of intervention which can be seen as neutral. Different theories may be applied to each method in its practical application. For example there can be very different types of individual work according to the theoretical orientation of the social worker, including psychodynamic individual work and task-centred work.

Social work approaches include such areas as community social work, feminist social work, radical social work, anti-racist approaches and citizen involvement and empowerment. They may be operationalised using a variety of methods drawing on diverse theoretical models. They are often distinguished by the social and political value base from which they draw.

Methods of social work intervention are informed by social work theories and their corresponding models. A good example of this is provided by Brown's models of group work: peer confrontation, problem-solving, task-centred, psychotherapeutic, self-help, human relations training and social goals (Brown, A. 1992). These models draw on a variety of social work theories and psychological ideas. The interrelationship of methods and theories is complex.

Within social work, particular theoretical approaches have dominated certain methods of intervention at specific times. The postwar period saw the predominance of psychodynamic theory within the method of individual counselling. Family work currently relies heavily on systems theory to engineer its direct intervention.

Social and political factors have been significant in the development of methods of intervention. Nowhere is this clearer than in the area of community work, where there has always been and there remains a debate between community development work and community activism (Dominelli, 1990; Ellis, 1989; Smith, 1989; Vass, 1979). In the former, the role of the community worker is to facilitate the creation of groups and communities to empower and help themselves; and in the latter the community worker takes on a far more explicit role in linking local community issues to their wider political contexts. Although the differences may have been inflated and criticisms have been levelled against the claim that community work can be politically active and effective within the British social structure (Vass, 1979), distinctions can still be drawn. The differences can be illustrated by looking at responses to, for example, racial harassment on a housing estate. The community development approach might involve helping residents experiencing harassment to organise a support group, to lessen feelings of isolation. How the support group might develop would be determined by its members. The community activist approach might involve the same initial steps, but there would then be more likelihood that the group would be directed towards making wider links both in their understanding of the harassment and its relationship to racism and in more proactive responses to it, informed by a particular political understanding and where necessary direct action to alter the structural context which breeds and feeds oppression.

At times, different methods of social work intervention are viewed in an exclusive manner. Agencies may be dominated by a particular method of intervention, irrespective of the nature of their referrals or the communities they serve. The most heavily relied on method has been, and still is, individual work. The nature of the referrals to social work agencies has meant that this has seemed the most appropriate and effective method of intervention. However, this is not always the case. Individual methods are often relied upon because they are the ones the agency is most familiar with providing and the methods that social workers are most comfortable practising; in a sense they are the most convenient, without regard to the needs of clients. This myopic approach may work against the interests of clients, reinforcing their isolation and feelings of disempowerment. As an illustration, the area social services team that the author of this chapter managed had a very high referral rate of single isolated people, who had periodic psychiatric difficulties. Traditionally the approach in the team had been to use individual work to support the person within the community, working with other agencies and services to prevent further hospitalisation. The community psychiatric nurses (CPNs) in the area took the same approach and the two agencies liaised closely with each other. It took the team some time to assess the limitations of their methods of intervention. Although some of the service users involved needed and benefited from individual methods, they might also have benefited from group work as a method of intervention. One social worker and a CPN were involved in the setting up of a group for these service users, starting as a problem-solving, task-centred group and developing into a self-help group. Some members of the group continued to need individual intervention, but the majority benefited from the group processes which helped break down the isolation which was often a contributory factor in individuals' mental health problems. The White City Project, which was set up to work with women experiencing depression, is an excellent example of how various methods of intervention can be brought together to enable the best possible outcome for users of a service (Holland, 1990).

Different methods of intervention offer varied possibilities; they all have their own benefits and limitations. It is important that serious thought is given to which method or combination of methods would be in the service users' interests.

*Processes involved in social work intervention*

Processes of social work intervention cover the area that is normally referred to as social work skills involved in direct work with people. This area is covered in Chapter 3. It appears briefly here because of the close interrelationship of knowledge and skills. Practitioners need to be familiar with the literature on skills and processes, as this is a central aspect of the knowledge base of social work. 'Processes involved in intervention' refers to the stages of engagement involved in direct work, from referral through to evaluation and review. Publications on community care offer helpful frameworks for thinking about the processes of all social work intervention, not only that relating to work with adults in need of services (Department of Health, 1991b; Smale et al., 1993).

Although the processes involved may differ to some extent, depending on the method of social work intervention and the context in which it takes place, there is a generic core of values (Chapter 2), and skills (Chapter 3) that are essential, whatever the context, to competent practice.

All three aspects – theories and their corresponding models, methods of intervention, and the processes involved in intervention – are the core of social work's knowledge base. However well social workers understand a client's situation and experience, if they cannot intervene in an informed and effective way they are of little use.

**Knowledge that clarifies the practitioner's understanding of
the legal, policy, procedural and organisational context in
which their practice takes place**

Social work does not operate in a vacuum: it is part of the complex
organisation of British society and the remaining structures of the
postwar welfare state. The roles and responsibilities of social work
are defined in a number of ways, but primarily through legislation
and related policies and procedures.

A working understanding of legislation, policies and procedures is
an essential component of the knowledge base of social work. It is
also the aspect of social work knowledge that practitioners often feel
most familiar with, particularly in relation to procedures. However,
it is this area that has often been highlighted in childcare inquiries as
the Achilles' heel of social work practice. Social workers have been
found to be ignorant of legislative and procedural structures or to
have misinterpreted and misused them (Department of Health,
1991b).

The use and understanding of law in social work practice is a
complex area, and one where there needs to be a close relationship
between knowledge and values. In most cases there are clear
guidelines for competent practice and the administration of law
particularly in childcare law, work with vulnerable adults, and
supervision of offenders. However, in view of the fact that social
work deals with difficult human issues, a rigid application of the law
divorced from other relevant considerations is inappropriate and as
an approach has drawn criticism (Butler-Sloss, 1988). There needs to
be reflective consideration of the relationship between law and social
work, to enable practitioners to work competently in the interests of
their clients (Braye and Preston-Shoot, 1990).

*The legislation*
Practitioners are often familiar with their own agencies' procedures
to facilitate the operation of some aspects of legislation, but remain
ignorant of the specific legislation itself. An example is the way
residential establishments for older people are referred to as Part III,
or assessments of older people are called Part III assessments. It is
not uncommon for social workers not to know that they are
referring to Part III of the National Assistance Act 1948, which
refers to the local authority's duty to provide residential accommodation to people who, by virtue of age, disability or other
circumstances, are considered to be in need of residential care.

As well as understanding that their intervention and service
delivery are directed by specific pieces of legislation, practitioners

need an understanding of the nature, sources and administration of the law (Ball, 1989). This involves knowledge of how legislation is formulated, enacted and administered. In addition social workers should be familiar with the jurisdiction of both criminal and civil courts and the operations of these courts.

There are few social work contexts in which welfare rights and housing advice work are not a significant part of a social worker's workload. This means that practitioners must constantly update their knowledge in these areas and be able to use appropriate advisory agencies effectively.

At the present time social work intervention and service delivery are organised into three broad categories that correspond to some degree with three pieces of legislation. Probation work is directly related to the Criminal Justice Act 1991; work with children and families relates to the Children Act 1989 and work with adults in need of support is covered primarily by the National Health Service and Community Care Act 1990. However, practice is not so simple. For example, adoption, although it has received attention in a White Paper (Department of Health, 1993c), still involves a complex range of laws and directives including the Adoption Act 1976; Adoption Rules 1984, the Adoption Agency Regulations 1983 and the Adoption (Amendment) Rules 1991. Social workers have to relate to Acts of Parliament or statutory rules which are constantly being amended, often on the basis of ideological shifts in government policy (for example the Criminal Justice and Public Order Act 1994 subverts many of the intentions of the Criminal Justice Act 1991 by questioning the capacity of community penalties to reform and control offenders).

This degree of complexity, which even lawyers find daunting, does not mean that social workers have to act as well-informed and trained specialist solicitors. This would not be desirable or possible. Rather the complexity points to the need for social workers to have a basic working knowledge of relevant legislation and to be on guard for changes in legal requirements and procedures in order to form a reliable body of knowledge that informs and guides, as far as professionally possible, their actions and the advice and guidance they give to service users. It is not possible for social workers to rely on their past knowledge. Past knowledge in legal terms may also mean 'outdated knowledge', and thus be dangerous. Social workers have a professional and moral duty constantly to familiarise themselves with the wider legal and political context of their work. This means updating their knowledge of the most recent legislation relevant to their tasks and duties, and pursuing, where necessary, 'refresher' courses (whether in-service or externally) to ensure that they keep in close touch with developments. Although the burden for this lies on the shoulders of every social worker, and failure or ignorance on their part is not excusable, this heavy responsibility is shared by their employers and trainers, who should offer opportunities for their staff to pursue such good practice. In many respects the failures and serious mistakes made by social workers, as identified in childcare inquiries, have much to do with both personal (social worker) and organisational (employer) failures to realise the need for regular training and familiarity with the legislation, procedures, and the roles of and powers vested in social workers.

CCETSW emphasises the importance of contextualising specific pieces of legislation to help the practitioner make sense of their relevance and use (Ball et al., 1991). The structure of this book reflects this, in as much as the legislation is placed in the context of particular areas of practice in the following chapters. Legislation and amendments to legislation is an interactive process which evolves through social policy initiatives and social, economic and political activity. Without referring to specific legislation it is possible to draw out some general points about social work's use of legal knowledge. First, there has to be a close relationship between values and knowledge. Social workers when carrying out their legal duties are involved in serious considerations of risk, restriction of liberty and removal. This necessitates the consideration of matters including discrimination, self-determination, empowerment and natural justice, to name but a few, if a practitioner is to invoke the law in an informed and constructive manner. Secondly, the practitioner needs to understand the social policy context of the legislation to appreciate its spirit and principles. Thirdly, statutes themselves are practically incomprehensible to anyone but a lawyer. White Papers, guidance and regulations relating to relevant legislation are both intelligible to non-lawyers and invaluable to social workers in facilitating an understanding of the legislation and clarifying its relevance to their practice. Fourthly, given that there are currently over fifty-one laws relevant to social work's roles and responsibilities (Ball et al., 1991:45), it is not realistic that practitioners should be acquainted with legislation other than that impacting on their work directly. Fifthly, social workers are not lawyers. There must be an effective working relationship between social workers and their legal departments or legal advisers. For this to be realised, they need a formal knowledge of the legal system and an informal knowledge of their own procedures for access to legal advice. Sixthly, competent practice in relation to the law means there needs to be competence in all three areas of knowledge, values and skills. For example, competence in court is essential, requiring a degree of confidence in the skills of giving evidence effectively, and knowledge of how courts function at both a formal and an informal level. Lastly, since legislation defines the roles and responsibilities of social work and the boundaries of welfare provision, this knowledge is essential for practitioners in whatever context their practice takes place.

*Policy and procedures*

Although we are governed by the same laws, whether we practise in Dolgellau or Islington, because law can be either mandatory or permissive, how it is interpreted in different settings varies. The complex relationship between local and central government means that varying emphasis is placed on laws by local authorities at different times. A Labour-controlled local authority might have difficulty implementing law that it sees as repressive and that has been enacted by a Conservative central government. This has been illustrated very clearly in the case of Section 28 of the Local Government Act 1988. Another example is the variety of ways assessment and care management have been arranged in different local authorities under the National Health Service and Community Care Act 1990 (Department of Health, 1993a). These variations necessitate a working knowledge of local government and its relationship to social work, and this has to be a component of the knowledge base of social work (Daniel and Wheeler, 1989).

Familiarity with the law, White Papers, guidance and regulation documents is essential for competent practice, but there are Department of Health, Home Office and Social Service Inspectorate publications that social workers need to keep pace with as well, as they are directly relevant to their work. Some social work agencies are systematic in their use of such documents. Probation officers, for example, will be familiar with *National Standards* (Home Office et al., 1992; 1995), as approved social workers are with the mental health *Code of Practice* (Department of Health, 1993b). However, regular reference to relevant texts of this nature is not uniform within social work.

Social work agencies are as complex organisations as the social issues they represent. Social workers, as well as having a working understanding of the law, legal guidance and processes, have the additional responsibility of gaining a knowledge of their own agency. This involves a practical knowledge of the agency's structure, how it is managed, and how the individual worker fits within the organisation; policies and procedures relevant to the social worker's context; roles and responsibilities; relationships to other relevant agencies and their operations, in terms of their structures, policies, procedures, provisions and personnel. This includes a working knowledge of agencies such as benefit agencies and housing departments, both essential to most social work practice. Lastly, they require knowledge of the day-to-day functioning of the agency, in order to operate efficiently and effectively.

Policies and procedures have often been developed within agencies to guarantee that standards of practice and provision do not fall below an acceptable level. In the same way that rigid application of the law has attracted criticism, so must we beware mindless following of agency procedures without full consideration of the circumstances of each unique situation.

Much of the knowledge outlined in this section will not be available in books, but will involve the practitioner in a proactive search to find out about their own work context. This is part of the bedrock of social work knowledge, and a very relevant part of competent practice.

*Organisational contexts*
Social work as a profession has always had some difficulty in defining exactly what it is, and indeed also in saying very succinctly what it does. This is not surprising, given the varied contexts in which it is expected to discharge its tasks and duties. It will only be possible to define what social work is in the particular context in which it takes place. Most social workers are primarily employees, which places them as professionals in a slightly different position than some other professional groups. The roles, tasks and responsibilities of social workers are often defined by the context in which they are employed, rather than being universally applicable to the profession as a whole.

The probation service, social services departments, hospitals, general practitioner surgeries, refugee organisations, psychotherapeutic communities, housing associations, community work settlements, self-help organisations, needle-exchange centres, adoption and fostering organisations, residential units, prisons, resource centres and community group homes are just a tiny selection of organisational contexts in which social work takes place. Practitioners must have a knowledge of their own agency's history, its remit, powers and functions, whether these are dictated by legislation or not, and how their agency fits within the overall picture of welfare provision.

Organisations have a habit of restructuring themselves from time to time. Social services reorganisation has become rather more than a habit. Restructuring of social work agencies has not always been either necessary in response to changing legislation or to do with bettering outcomes for service users. Changes are often instigated on political grounds and in an attempt to manage growing demands and the resulting increase in anxiety (Brown and Pearce, 1992). Practitioners, to remain useful, need to have an understanding of organisational change, its causes, and strategies for survival. Social work finds itself in uncertain times, with individual workers and their agencies having to manage an unprecedented degree of imposed changes. Some of these changes have been of great benefit, but have necessitated a fresh analysis of social work's future. The decreasing size of the statutory sector and the increasing role of the voluntary and independent service provider sector (with fewer resources), has meant that much assumed knowledge about organisations' roles and functions has to be rethought. This requires an awareness of current changes that may impact on the functions of practitioners within agencies. Social workers must understand their new role and position in the social structure of their agency as well as society, and at the same time work out how they can adjust and adapt themselves and their practices to the changes.

## Conclusion: competence and knowledge

Despite the multi-faceted nature of social work with all its varied responsibilities and tasks, sometimes seemingly unrelated, it is still possible to define what practitioners in a generic sense need as part of their knowledge base. Whatever the setting, practitioners need the three components of knowledge outlined in this chapter to work efficiently: knowledge that informs the practitioner about the client's experience and context; knowledge that helps the practitioner plan appropriate intervention; and knowledge that clarifies the practitioner's understanding of the legal, policy, procedural and organisational context in which their practice takes place. Knowledge is only one aspect of competence; values and skills are also essential. For knowledge to be useful to practice, there needs to be a solid integration of all three.

> 'Knowledge must be treated as a constant, dynamic process of being. That is to say, it is evolutionary. It has a social career of its own. It is constantly expanded, defined, and redefined according to changes in the sociopolitical, moral and economic characteristics of a particular society during a particular period by particular governments and by particular individuals and groups. In that form, knowledge is a constant companion that has to be negotiated, accommodated and transcended to deal with new situations. Social workers must treat knowledge as a transactional process. Social life and problems in social relationships (which are the subject matter of social work) are not static. They are ever changing.' (Vass, 1987)

Social work knowledge must be seen in the same way: as a constantly evolving core of ideas which are translated into praxis by flexible, competent and reflective practitioners.

## References

Ahmad, B. (1990) *Black Perspectives in Social Work.* Birmingham: Venture Press.

Ahmed, S. (1994) 'Anti-racist social work: a black perspective', in C. Hanvey and T. Philpot (eds), *Practising Social Work.* London: Routledge. pp. 119–33.

Ball, C. (1989) *Law for Social Workers: An Introduction.* Aldershot: Wildwood House.

Ball, C., Roberts, G., Trench, S. and Vernon, S. (1991) *Teaching, Learning and Assessing Social Work Law.* London: CCETSW.

Bandura, A. (1977) *Social Learning Theory.* Englewood Cliffs, NJ: Prentice-Hall.

Barker, M. and Hardiker, P. (eds) (1981) *Theories of Practice in Social Work.* London: Academic Press.

Barrett, M. and McIntosh, M. (1982) *The Anti-Social Family.* London: Verso.

Beresford, P. and Croft, S. (1993) *Citizen Involvement. A Practical Guide for Change.* Basingstoke: Macmillan.

Berger, R.M. (1990) 'Older gays and lesbians', in R.J. Kus, (ed.), *Keys to Caring: Assisting Your Gay and Lesbian Clients.* Boston: Alyson Publications. pp. 170–81.

Bowlby, J. (1988) *A Secure Base: Clinical Applications of Attachment Theory.* London: Routledge.

Brake, M. and Bailey, R. (eds) (1980) *Radical Social Work and Practice.* London: Edward Arnold.

Braye, S. and Preston-Shoot, M. (1990) 'On teaching and applying the law in social work: it is not that simple', *British Journal of Social Work,* 20(4): 333–53.

Brown, A. (1992) *Groupwork,* 3rd edn. Aldershot: Avebury.

Brown, H.C. (1991) 'Competent child-focused practice: working with lesbian and gay carers', *Adoption and Fostering,* 15(2): 11–17.

Brown, H.C. (1992a) 'Gender, sex and sexuality in the assessment of prospective carers', *Adoption and Fostering,* 16(2): 30–34.

Brown, H.C. (1992b) 'Lesbians, the state and social work practice', in M. Langan and L. Day (eds), *Women, Oppression and Social Work.* London: Routledge. pp. 201–19.

Brown, H.C. and Pearce, J.J. (1992) 'Good practice in the face of anxiety: social work with girls and young women', *Journal of Social Work Practice,* 6(2): 159–65.

Bryan, A. (1992) 'Working with black single mothers: myths and reality', in M. Langan and L. Day (eds), *Women, Oppression and Social Work.* London: Routledge. pp. 169–85.

Burck, C. and Speed, B. (1995) *Gender, Power and Relationships.* London: Routledge.

Burrell, G. and Morgan, G. (1979) *Sociological Paradigms and Organisational Analysis.* London: Heinemann.

Butler-Sloss, E. (1988) *Report of the Enquiry into Child Abuse in Cleveland.* London: HMSO.

Carew, R. (1979) 'The place of knowledge in social work activity', *British Journal of Social Work,* 9(3): 349–64.

CCETSW (1989) *Improving Standards in Practice Learning.* London: Central Council for Education and Training in Social Work.

CCETSW (1991) *DipSW: Rules and Requirements for the Diploma in Social Work*, 2nd edn. London: Central Council for Education and Training in Social Work.

Channer, Y. and Parton, N. (1990) 'Racism, cultural relativism and child protection', in The Violence Against Children Study Group (ed.), *Taking Child Abuse Seriously*. London: Unwin Hyman. pp. 105–20.

Clare, A. (1980) *Psychiatry in Dissent*. London: Tavistock.

Coulshed, V. (1991) *Social Work Practice. An Introduction*, 2nd edn. Basingstoke: Macmillan.

Daniel, P. and Wheeler, J. (1989) *Social Work and Local Politics*. Basingstoke: Macmillan.

Department of Health (1991a) *Assessment and Care Management*. London: HMSO.

Department of Health (1991b) *Child Abuse. A Study of Inquiry Reports, 1980–1989*. London: HMSO.

Department of Health (1993a) *Inspection of Assessment and Care Management Arrangements in Social Services Departments*. London: HMSO.

Department of Health (1993b) *Code of Practice: Mental Health Act 1983*. London: HMSO.

Department of Health (1993c) *Adoption: The Future*, cm 2288. London: HMSO.

Dominelli, L. (1988) *Anti-racist Social Work*. Basingstoke: Macmillan.

Dominelli, L. (1990) *Women and Community Action*. Birmingham: Venture Press.

Dominelli, L. and McLeod, E. (1989) *Feminist Social Work*. Basingstoke: Macmillan.

Downes, D. and Rock, P. (1988) *Understanding Deviance: A Guide to the Sociology of Crime and Rule Breaking*, 2nd edn. Oxford: Oxford University Press.

Eichenbaum, L. and Orbach, S. (1983) *Understanding Women*. Harmondsworth: Penguin.

Ellis, J. (1989) *Breaking New Ground: Community Development with Asian Communities*. London: Bedford Square Press.

Erikson, E. (1965) *Childhood and Society*, 2nd edn. London: Hogarth Press.

Ernst, S. and Maguire, M. (eds) (1987) *Living with the Sphinx*. London: The Women's Press.

Goffman, E. (1961) *Asylums*. Harmondsworth: Penguin.

Hall, A. and Fagen, R. (1956) 'Definition of system', in *General Systems Year Book I*. pp. 18–28. (Revised paper first presented at *Systems Engineers*, a course at Bell Telephone Laboratories. New York: Bell Telephone Laboratories).

Hanmer, J. and Statham, D. (1988) *Women and Social Work*. Basingstoke: Macmillan.

Hanvey, C. and Philpot, T. (eds) (1994) *Practising Social Work*. London: Routledge.

Heder, P., Duncan, S. and Gray, M. (1993) *Beyond Blame: Child Abuse Tragedies Revisited*. London: Routledge.

Holland, S. (1990) 'Psychotherapy, oppression and social action: gender, race and class in black women's depression', in R.J. Perelberg and A.C. Miller (eds), *Gender and Power in Families*. London: Tavistock/Routledge. pp. 256–69.

Home Office, Department of Health and Welsh Office (1992) *National Standards for the Supervision of Offenders in the Community*. London: HMSO.

Home Office, Department of Health and Welsh Office (1995) *National Standards for the Supervision of Offenders in the Community*. London: HMSO.

Howe, D. (1986) 'The segregation of women and their work in the personal social services', *Critical Social Policy*, 5(3): 21–35.

Howe, D. (1987) *An Introduction to Social Work Theory*. Aldershot: Wildwood House.

Hudson, A. with Ayensu, L., Oadley, C. and Patocchi, M. (1994) 'Practising feminist approaches', in C. Hanvey and T. Philpot (eds), *Practising Social Work*. London: Routledge. pp. 93–105.

Husband, C. (1991) 'Race, conflictual politics, and anti-racist social work: lessons from the past for action in the '90s', in C.D. Project Steering Group, *Setting the Context for Change*. Leeds: CCETSW. pp. 46–73.

Hutchinson-Reis, M. (1989) 'And for those of us who are blacks? Black politics in social work', in M. Langan and P. Lee (eds), *Radical Social Work Today*. London: Unwin Hyman. pp. 165–77.

Jordan, B. and Parton, N. (1983) *The Political Dimension of Social Work*. Oxford: Basil Blackwell.

Kubler-Ross, E. (1973) *On Death and Dying*. Basingstoke: Macmillan.

Langan, M. and Day, L. (eds) (1992) *Women, Oppression and Social Work*. London: Routledge.

Langan, M. and Lee, P. (eds) (1989) *Radical Social Work Today*. London: Unwin Hyman.

Lawrence, M. (1992) 'Women's psychology and feminist social work practice', in M. Langan and L. Day (eds), *Women, Oppression and Social Work*. London: Routledge. pp. 31–47.

Lindermann, E. (1944) 'Symptomatology and management of acute grief', in H.J. Parad (ed.), *Crisis Intervention: Selected Readings*. New York: Family Service Association of America. pp. 7–21.

Lishman, J. (ed.) (1991) *Handbook of Theory for Practice Teachers in Social Work*. London: Jessica Kingsley.

London Borough of Brent (1985) *A Child in Trust. Report on the Death of Jasmine Beckford*. London: London Borough of Brent.

London Borough of Lambeth (1987) *Whose Child? The Report of the Panel Appointed to Inquire into the Death of Tyra Henry*. London: London Borough of Lambeth.

Maclean, M. and Groves, D. (1991) *Women's Issues in Social Policy*. London: Routledge.

MacLeod, M. and Saraga, E. (1987) *Child Sexual Abuse: Towards a Feminist Professional Practice*. London: Polytechnic of North London Press.

Mayer, E.J. and Timms, N. (1970) *The Client Speaks*. London: Routledge & Kegan Paul.

Nicholson, P. and Bayne, R. (1990) *Applied Psychology for Social Workers*, 2nd edn. Basingstoke: Macmillan.

O'Hagan, K. (1986) *Crisis Intervention in Social Services*. Basingstoke: Macmillan.

Oliver, M. (1991) *Social Work, Disabled People and Disabling Environments*. London: Jessica Kingsley.

Parad, H.J. (ed.) (1965) *Crisis Intervention: Selected Readings*. New York, Family Service Association of America.

Parkes, C.M. (1972) *Bereavement: Studies of Grief in Adult Life*. New York: International Universities Press.

Parton, N. (1985) *The Politics of Child Abuse*. Basingstoke: Macmillan.

Payne, M. (1991) *Modern Social Work Theory*. Basingstoke: Macmillan.

Payne, M. (1992) 'Psychodynamic theory within the politics of social work theory', *Journal of Social Work Practice*, 6(2): 141–9.

Pearson, G. (1975) *The Deviant Imagination*. Basingstoke: Macmillan.

Pearson, G., Treseder, J. and Yelloly, M. (1988) *Social Work and the Legacy of Freud*. Basingstoke: Macmillan.

Perelberg, R.J. and Miller, A.C. (eds) (1990) *Gender and Power in Families*. London: Routledge.

Phoenix, A. (1990) 'Theories of gender and black families', in T. Lovell (ed.) *British Feminist Thought*. Oxford: Blackwell. pp. 119–33.

Piaget, J. (1952) *The Origins of Intelligence in Children*. New York: International Universities Press.

Pilalis, J. and Anderton, J. (1986) 'Feminism and family therapy', *Journal of Family Therapy*, 9(2): 99–113.

Pincus, A. and Minahan, A. (1973) *Social Work Practice: Model and Method*. Itasca, IL: F.E. Peacock.

Robertson, J. and Robertson, J. (1989) *Separation and the Very Young*. London: Free Association Books.

Rojek, C. (1986) 'The "subject" in social work', *British Journal of Social Work*, 16(2): 65–77.

Rojek, C., Peacock, G. and Collins, C. (1988) *Social Work and Received Ideas*. London: Routledge.

Ryburn, M. (1991) 'The myth of assessment', *Adoption and Fostering*, 15(1): 20–27.

Scull, A.T. (1984) *Decarcerations: Community Treatment and the Deviant: A Radical View*, 2nd edn. Cambridge: Basil Blackwell/Polity Press.

Sheldon, B. (1978) 'Theory and practice in social work: a re-examination of a tenuous relationship', *British Journal of Social Work*, 8(1): 1–22.

Smale, G. and Tuson, G. with Biehal, N. and Marsh, P. (1993) *Empowerment, Assessment, Care Management and the Skilled Worker*. London: HMSO.

Smith, I. (1989) 'Community work in recession: a practitioner's perspective', in M. Langan and P. Lee (eds), *Radical Social Work Today*. London: Unwin Hyman. pp. 258–78.

Specht, H. and Vickery, A. (eds ) (1977) *Integrating Social Work Methods*. London: Allen & Unwin.

Statham, D. (1978) *Radicals in Social Work*. London: Routledge & Kegan Paul.

Stenson, K. and Gould, N. (1986) 'A comment on "A Framework for Theory in Social Work"' by Whittington and Holland, *Issues in Social Work Education*, 6(1): 41–5.

Thompson, N. (1993) *Anti-discriminatory Practice*. Basingstoke: Macmillan.

Tsoi, M. and Yule, J. (1982) 'Building up new behaviours: shaping, prompting and fading', in W. Yule and J. Carr (eds), *Behaviour Modification for the Mentally Handicapped*. London: Croom Helm.

Vass, A.A. (1979) 'The myth of a radical trend in British community work: a comparison between statutory and voluntary projects', *Community Development Journal*, 14: 3–13.

Vass, A.A. (1984) *Sentenced to Labour: Close Encounters with a Prison Substitute*. St Ives: Venus Academica.

Vass, A.A. (1986) *AIDS: A Plague in Us: A Social Perspective. The Condition and its Social Consequences*. St Ives: Venus Academica.

Vass, A.A. (1987) 'Sociology and social work', lecture notes, *Social Problems and Social Policy*, School of Social Work and Health Services. London: Middlesex University.

Vass, A.A. (1990) *Alternatives to Prison: Punishment, Custody and the Community*. London: Sage.

Violence Against Children Study Group (1990) *Taking Child Abuse Seriously*. London: Unwin Hyman.

Wilson, E. (1977) *Women and the Welfare State*. London: Tavistock.

Winnicott, C. (1964) *Child Care and Social Work*. Hitchin: Codicote Press.

Worden, W.J. (1983) *Grief Counselling and Grief Therapy*. London: Tavistock/ Routledge.

Yelloly, M.A. (1980) *Social Work Theory and Psychoanalysis*. London: Van Nostrand Reinhold.

# 2

# The Values of Social Work

> the basic assumption is that there is no value-free way of working in the
> welfare state, or indeed of living one's life, and that a person entrusted to
> some extent with other people's lives has obligations both to know his or
> her own values and their significance in action, and to be able to
> understand some of the forces in society that deeply and dramatically
> affect values in general. (Hardy, 1981: vii)

Ten years later, the Central Council for the Education and Training
of Social Workers (CCETSW, 1991a:15) argued thus:

> competence in social work practice requires the understanding and
> integration of the values of social work.

This continuing emphasis on values reflects concern from individuals
and government-sponsored bodies to identify the core values that
underpin social work practice (Clark and Asquith, 1985:1).

For social work practice to work with its dual mandate, delivering
care while exercising control, individual practitioners must accommodate central social work values to guide their professional
judgement. Core contradictions can exist in the aim to deliver a non-
oppressive, empowering practice while simultaneously defining and
controlling socially unacceptable behaviour: where the role of the
social worker fluctuates between defending society's values to
defending the client against the oppressive dominant values which
undermine individual choice and liberty (Cypher, 1975; Brown,
1992; Dominelli, 1988:121).

But what are social work values and how do they affect competences in social work practice? In this chapter we address these
two questions first by placing the discussion of values within the
context of the present political climate. Secondly, we examine the
increasing awareness of the importance of a critical examination of
social work values. Such analysis shows that 'values' have been on
the social work agenda since the 1890s. Recognising the integral
relationship between theory and practice as it changes through
history provides scope for an analysis of praxis. This comprises both
reflection and action which helps to prevent theory from being
divorced from actual events. It is through such analysis that we can

recognise the way that values are embedded in a fluid and changing social work practice.

Thirdly, we draw on definitions of core values to social work practice, referring to the characteristics of demonstrated values by addressing specific terms such as 'freedom of and respect for the individual', 'self-determination', 'freedom from oppression and negative discrimination' (CCETSW, 1991a:15), or as described in the amended requirements: 'identify, analyse and take action to counter discrimination, racism, disadvantage, inequality and injustice' (CCETSW, 1995:4). The application of these values in practice places the power relationships between practitioner and client as central concerns in social work intervention. The multi-faceted nature of social work and relevant legislation is addressed to illustrate how the roles and tasks facing social work practitioners create different moral conflicts. While defined values exist as absolute truths, their application in practice must recognise the diverse and specific circumstances of individual experience.

Finally, we conclude by stressing the importance of the social worker's awareness of self: the ontological nature of personal values and their effect on professional judgements. Through working towards knowing and owning fears, aspirations and values, individual workers can extend the systemic analysis of power between individuals to make connections between themselves, their profession and the local community they serve (Conn and Turner, 1990).

## The political context of social work values

The plethora of definitions of 'traditional values' that followed the call for 'back to basics' from the Conservative Party during 1993 highlights the difficulty inherent in asserting commonly shared, core values across a fragmented and divided society. The neo-liberal consumer-led politics of the 1990s which places importance on the strength and survival of the individual is prevalent throughout much of contemporary British society. The plea for 'back to basics' from the present Right is asserting a contradictory voice in the consumer-led wilderness for some sense of moral standards, some value distinction between right and wrong to exist while individuals battle for economic survival. Such pleas have been reinforced by the genuine despair caused by a number of recent cases, often involving children who personify a future society where moral rules and social values have been destroyed. The 'joy riders'' threatening and challenging behaviour (Campbell, 1993) and the shock of the unimaginable behaviour in the James Bulger case are but two examples which raise questions of where the family, school, Church and state have responsibility in distinguishing between acceptable and unacceptable behaviour. Although work by Pearson (1983) shows us that the 'good old days' were not such a safe haven of goodwill, and Vass (1986) shows us that moral panics occur at regular intervals throughout the course of history, there are specific ramifications of these concerns in the 1990s. The onus on instilling individual responsibility within the adult population ranges from the emphasis placed by business schools on 'ethics in business', to the suggestion that the state invest £2.1 million in leafleting households in a desperate attempt to inform adults of their tasks and responsibilities in child-rearing (Meikle, 1994:3). Contemporary politics mourns the demise of the socially responsible individual and looks to a revival of values of the past to rectify the apparent present morass.

While the Right attempts to assert some order through its plea for 'back to basics', the Left questions the 'master narratives' that have underpinned the moral truths and values of the past. For example, the relevance of historically located values, embedded within the traditional working class, to the technological workforce of the 1990s is questioned. Similarly, the value base of established representative political movements has been seen to exclude specific individuals. The socialist movement has been seen to focus on the white male worker (Rowbotham et al., 1979), while the feminist movement has failed to accommodate the multi-faceted nature of discriminatory politics that separates black women, lesbians, older women and women with disabilities from each other (Langan and Day, 1992; Spelman, 1988). Developing sociological theory recognises this fragmentation by placing importance on the ontological prefiguration of self in a diverse political arena. Emphasis is now being placed on the way that individuals define themselves and their relationship to representative political movements (Probyn, 1993; Foucault, 1991; Seidler, 1991:65; Yelloly, 1993). The central, assumed universal values of the Left as a representative party are being attacked. Both the individualistic, right-wing consumerism and the left-wing postmodernism threaten the myth of the stability of previously accepted values (Mercer, 1990).

Despite this, there is a strong body of theory outlining social work's commitment to commonly held values (Clark and Asquith, 1985; CCETSW, 1991a, 1995; Payne, 1991; Peacock and Collins, 1989; Shardlow, 1989). Within the increasingly articulated social turmoil of the 1990s, progressive moves have been made to assert basic values that underpin social work practice. According to the Central Council for Education and Training in Social Work

(CCETSW, 1991a:15; see also CCETSW, 1995) qualifying social workers should have a commitment to the following aspirations:

- the value and dignity of individuals;
- the right to respect, privacy and confidentiality;
- the right of individuals and families to choose;
- the strengths and skills embedded in local communities.

Recent legislation has incorporated such objectives. For example, the Children Act 1989 requires that consideration be taken of individual need and circumstance: the child and those with parental responsibility must be given full opportunity to be involved in decision-making processes (Home Office, 1991:1). Regard is to be given to the child's racial and cultural needs and to the strengths of extended family and community networks (Children Act 1989: schedule 2 para. 11). Community Care legislation (National Health Service and Community Care Act 1990) has the central premise that the strengths of the local community be respected, and that people have the right to be cared for within their own community; The Criminal Justice Act 1991 notes the need to avoid discrimination on the grounds of race, sex or any other improper ground (Criminal Justice Act 1991: schedule 95 (1) (b)). Although social work does not occur in isolation from the political, geographical and economic climate, it has maintained a professional momentum which defines and asserts values central to its role in the delivery of competent practice.

We discuss below the origins of these values, which have developed through a political and historical process. We then move to look at the complexities of applying them to a social work practice which recognises the needs of the individual within a diverse and competing society.

**The historical context of values in social work**

To place the current situation in context it is helpful to explore the origins of social work values in theory and in practice.

It is no coincidence that the present call for a return to traditional values is accompanied both by a reduction in state resources for social work practice and by a proliferation of the number of charitable organisations working in the caring sector. Harker (1992:192) shows how the income of charitable organisations has dramatically increased over the last decade, while others express concern that some of them are being asked to plug the gaps left by changes and diminutions in government funding (Carter et al., 1992). This emphasis on the role of charitable organisations coincides with the promotion of the nuclear family as provider for individual need. The recent newsworthy scapegoating of single mothers as scroungers on state resources causing the fragmentation of the nuclear family (Moore, 1993) shows a desperate attempt to isolate the demise of traditional nuclear family values as the cause of all society's ills. Such work detracts attention from the well researched issues of poverty and poor health experienced by a range of family groups throughout the country: issues which highlight the stress on individuals and households in their attempts to sustain health and well-being without having to become dependent upon diminishing state resources (Blackburn, 1991; Glendinning and Millar, 1992).

Self-reliance and self-determination were originally promoted through charitable acts as opposed to state intervention. The role of the voluntary, charitable organisation was advanced in the late 1800s. As Woodroofe (1962:32) observes: 'true charity administered according to certain principles could encourage independence, strengthen character and help to preserve the family as the fundamental unit of society'. Charitable relief was to enhance independence and strength of character. This became overt with the advent of the industrial revolution, which appeared to be creating a divided society: the upper and middle classes gaining financial benefit from the industrial developments while large fragments of the working class lived in increasing poverty and 'outside the prosperity and political pale' (Woodroofe, 1962:6).

Voicing concern for the welfare of the individual in the midst of increasing poverty, General William Booth made a plea for the dignity and autonomy of the individual by advocating the extension of the Cab Horse charter. 'When a horse is down it be helped up, when it lives it has food, shelter and work' (Booth, 1890:18). Booth asked for respect and dignity to be extended to all people. He argued that many were denied this right. Laying the foundation for Beveridge to claim that 'want' was needless (Beveridge, 1942), Booth reflected the middle-class consciousness which spurred the philanthropic foundation of the Charity Organisation Society (COS) in 1869. The COS, representing some 640 institutions from London alone, regulated the expenditure of relief to the poor, while it aimed to increase the moral structure of the individual and society. It was believed that charity, administered according to certain principles, could 'encourage independence, strengthen character and help to preserve the family as the fundamental unit of society' (Woodroofe, 1962:32).

The conflict between the role of the state and charitable organisations became identified by an increasing awareness of poverty as a measurable concern defined by the Poor Laws (1834). This conflict spurred debate about the value and purpose of relief from the state to the poor, a relief which many felt inhibited the development of personal autonomy and voluntary action. The conflict was addressed in Beveridge's clarification of the roles and tasks of state intervention (Beveridge, 1942).

*Critical analysis of covert values: radical social work within the liberal democracy*
Radical social work of the postwar era made an essential connection between the donation of financial relief and the building of 'moral' character, making it clear that relief had hitherto rarely been delivered at random. It was argued that the values of middle-class life were being taught to the poor, who were categorised as either deserving or undeserving of future support (Bailey and Brake, 1975:5). The radical social work tradition challenged this polarisation of the 'undeserving' against the deserving poor, and the subsequent discrepancies in the provision of financial support. They argued that the individual's good health and welfare was being maintained not for humanitarian reasons but because it was essential to the survival of the liberal democracy: as the industrial revolution needed a healthy and compliant workforce, the social structure responded by promoting shared values to create social solidarity. The liberal democracy promoted its well-being through calming and containing group political unrest: angry or disaffected workers were isolated from each other through the advent of individualised casework, enhanced by the promotion of psychoanalytical theories in the 1970s (Bailey and Brake, 1975:4–8). According to Bailey and Brake (1975:6): 'Social problems became individualised, and the profession became immersed in an ideology which devalued political action.'

This critical perspective advanced by the radical social work tradition challenged philanthropic middle-class values. Scope was identified for social work practice to become part of a revolutionary mechanism for bringing about social change by advancing the interests of an oppressed working class.

This emphasis draws on theories of praxis which have their routes in Hegelian theory interpreted by Marxists such as Lukacs (1971). These theories argue that the dominant values and ideologies become internalised by individuals, who then develop a false consciousness of their value within society, a value determined by their status as workers within the labour market. The inherent internal frictions for the individual provide scope for what Mannheim (1948) argued to be an objective mind: individuals develop awareness of their relationship to the capitalist society. Radical social work saw the potential for social work to enhance individuals' awareness of their internalisation of the dominant values of the state. Instead of charitable donations pacifying the disaffected by extending dominant, middle-class values, radical social work argued that state resources could be used to empower individuals to recognise the potential for change.

Dismissed as romantic idealism by some (Davies, 1985: 3–15), such an approach introduces a critical analysis of the covert values of social work practice. It asks for the individual situated in opposition to the dominant ideology to be identified not as a problem, but as the locus within which inherent contradictions that exist throughout society are enacted. Without such recognition, the individual challenging covert values is open to being labelled as a deviant or a delinquent. For example, as Gilroy (1987:11) suggests, 'the idea that blacks comprise a problem, or more accurately a series of problems, is today expressed at the core of racist reasoning'.

As the core nature of oppression is its capacity to establish 'deviant' or 'problematic' individuals or groups falling outside the reasoning of the dominant value base as alien entities, we realise the importance of identifying the values behind practice. It is through the attempt to identify and reveal hidden value assumptions that a non-judgmental service can evolve. The radical social work tradition criticised the emergence of psychodynamic therapeutic interventions with the individual which emerged during the 1970s. It argued that the dominant middle-class value base of such practice remained unquestioned. Individual clients were seen to be pathologised, separated and isolated from their collective working-class roots. Such debate fed into an increasingly critical analysis of the role for psychodynamic theory within social work practice at the time (Pearson et al., 1988).

However, critics of the radical social work tradition argued that the rights of the individual could be overlooked through an analysis which assumed groups of individuals to share common properties. The assumption that middle and working class individuals shared common values, and that the casework approach with the individual could not provide the arena for empowerment to take place, was questioned. Enhanced by the feminist, anti-racist and other movements of the 1970s, differences within class categories were exposed (Cheetham, 1981; Dominelli, 1988). While such political movements were informed by and contributed to the radical social work tradition, there was a concurrent emphasis on addressing the interface between forms of oppression.

More recent sociological and social work theory extended this analysis to recognise diversity of individual need. For example, the increasing awareness of culture and ethnicity during the 1970s and 1980s invariably isolated culture as the central dimension to the client and worker encounter. The individual client, however, may identify 'culture' as only one of many multi-faceted and interconnected dimensions of themselves. Similarly, the needs and interests of individual gays or lesbians were grouped together into a common identity. Homophobic society located sexual behaviour as the defining characteristic of identity, but, as argued by Brown, 'reality, not surprisingly, is more complex' (1992:202). The ability of individual lesbians to parent successfully has been tainted by a number of prejudiced myths. Despite psychiatric and psychological research disproving the myths, Brown (1992:214) notes the need for an improvement in service which requires social workers to 'assess those individuals and their unique situation, and not rely on prejudiced assumptions'.

### Valuing the individual

This more recent emphasis on the difference and diversity of individual experience echoes a client-centred practice which starts from 'where the client is at'. The client-centred approach asks that the individual be respected as a human being, with specific needs and interests that cannot be generalised or assumed (Payne, 1991:24).

It was Beistek's work which aimed to separate the individual as a human being worthy of respect from his or her actions (Beistek, 1965). The need for respect for the individual, enhanced by humanist and existential models of social psychology (Rogers, 1951, 1961; Maslow, 1970), informed the development of individual client-centred counselling work. Roger's development of the client, or 'person-centred' therapy assumed that workers are 'genuine and congruent', can display 'unconditional positive regard' for their clients and can 'empathise' with the clients' view of the world (Payne, 1991: 169–70).

Incorporating theory from the client-centred approach, arguments for an anti-discriminatory practice have claimed that differences between clients must be recognised and acknowledged. This presents a direct challenge to practitioners who may feel inclined to make assumptions about an individual because of their race, sex, sexual orientation, class, age or ability. For Payne (1991:24), individualism is therefore 'not only an important value, it is significant for technical reasons'.

Individualism respects the scope for clients to take responsibility for their actions. Recognising and owning a problem as yours makes it become easier to take self-determined steps to address it. Instead of only being told what the problem looks like to others, the client identifies what the problem looks like to himself/herself. This aims to engage clients in actively identifying and addressing their behaviour. The complex forms of power-sharing and self-exploration that emerge from attempts to peel away assumption and myth are explored in much of the more recent literature on power and empowerment (Ward and Mullender, 1991; Page, 1992).

*The CCETSW strategy*

A number of developments contributed to the issues raised above being addressed by the Central Council for Education and Training (CCETSW) during the late 1980s and early 1990s. First, the increasing awareness of the need for practice to challenge negative discrimination was made overt (Ahmed et al., 1986; Oliver, 1990; Dominelli, 1988; Dominelli and McLeod, 1989). Secondly, concerns around social work competences within the field of child protection were prompted by the range of child abuse inquiries since 1974 (Department of Health, 1991a). Finally, the development of the Diploma in Social Work and of the accreditation of pre- and post-qualifying courses demanded that core values be clearly articulated and explained. The subsequent CCETSW strategy included publication of a number of documents which provided guidelines for social work training and practice, outlining core knowledge, skills and values. *CCETSW Paper 30* (CCETSW, 1991a) was accompanied by a number of publications in the 'Improving Social Work Education and Training' series, which consider a range of models of good practice. Common to all is the recognition that good, competent practice is reflected in workers' analysis of both the covert and overt assumptions of political categories, of their own personal and professional relationship to these categories, and of the specific needs and interests of the individual client. This is reflected in the CCETSW statement (CCETSW, 1991a:15) that social work values reflect 'a commitment to social justice and social welfare, to enhancing the quality of life of individuals, families and groups within communities, and to a repudiation of all forms of negative discrimination' (see also CCETSW, 1995:4).

**Social work values in practice**

In this section we apply social work values as identified by CCETSW to social work practice. Notwithstanding criticisms levelled at attempts to produce exhaustive lists of 'values' which will inevitably exclude some important considerations such as 'flexibility' and 'blame' (Timms and Timms, 1977:183), there are specific core values which form the basis of the development of competent practice.

First we explore the rights attributed to the individual, considering implications for childcare practice in general, and for working within current childcare legislation (Children Act 1989) in particular. Secondly, we look at the value placed on the strengths, skills and expertise within the local community of which the individual is a part. With this in mind we consider 'participation and self-help' as values respected within community care legislation (National Health Service and Community Care Act 1990). Thirdly, we address the role of the social worker in demonstrating a commitment to social justice and social welfare through an analysis of the nature of social work with offenders under the Criminal Justice Act 1991, with 1993 amendments.

We argue throughout this book that while absolute values can be used as a premise for the development of practice, the strength of social work practice is in the identification and challenge of various forms of negative discrimination, and in the acknowledgement of difference and diversity between the needs and interests of individual clients.

The social work values outlined below are transferable across different forms of practice. While they are described in relation to specific legislation and areas of practice, they are applicable to different forms of social work intervention with a range of client groups.

## The rights of the individual: with specific reference to childcare

Value is placed on the dignity of individuals, their right to respect, privacy and confidentiality, their right to protection from abuse, exploitation and violence. Individuals and their family have a right to choose, while the strengths and skills of local communities are to be respected (CCETSW, 1991a:15).

## The right to freedom from harm or abuse

A core value of social work theory and practice is the expectation that the individual has a right to freedom from harm or abuse. This right also extends to the protection of others, the community in general, from the individual's or group's harmful behaviour. With regard to the individual, it encompasses the expectation that those in positions of authority – parents, carers and professional workers – will not abuse the power invested in them (Department of Health, 1991b; CCETSW, 1991a, 1991b, 1991c).

With respect to childcare this applies to ensuring that the child's needs and wishes are respected and that his/her welfare is considered to be of paramount importance (Children Act 1989: section 1(1)). The complexities around the triangular relationship of child, carer and professional are revealed in the context of 'partnership' (Macdonald, 1991). This requires the views and circumstances of the client to be considered and respected, with an awareness of power differentials between client and worker. Lessons from two inquiries into child protection, the Beckford and Cleveland inquiries (London Borough of Brent, 1985; Department of Health and Social Security, 1988, respectively) give practical illustrations of the damage caused when parents, carers or social work agencies abuse the power entrusted in them. The concern in the Beckford case was that the parents' abuse of power against the child was not challenged by statutory authorities; and concern from the Cleveland case was that the relevant professional agencies abused their power by failing to respect the parents' right to information and consultation (Department of Health and Social Security, 1988). These two brief examples help to emphasise the complexities involved when using authority, entrusted to the worker, to ensure that the child's right to 'good enough' parenting is protected (CCETSW, 1991d:32).

Central to the existence of the right to protection is the maintenance of accountable and recorded communication between those involved. Although in situations of conflict of interest between parent and child, the child's interest must be given first consideration (Department of Health, 1991b:9; Children Act 1989: section 1(1)), parents have the right to 'an open and honest approach'; the right to have their 'own views sought'; the right to have the scope to 'challenge information held on them and decisions taken that affect them'; the right to 'careful assessment'; and the right to have the workers' statutory duties explained to them (Department of Health, 1991b:9, 11). The Department of Health and Social Security's report (1988) of the Inquiry into Child Abuse in Cleveland illustrates the pitfalls in not upholding these values. It demonstrates how legal proceedings were advanced without due consideration of the merits of each case, and without a proper recognition of parental rights as outlined above (Payne, 1991:25).

Adults should have their rights respected, but valuing the individual does not mean condoning all and any behaviour (CCETSW, 1991d:92–3). The worker reserves his/her statutory duty to protect the child from significant harm (Children Act 1989: section 31). It is essential that assessment must continue to be 'promoting the safety and well being of the child' (Department of Health, 1991b:13). The potential for 'dangerousness' arises, therefore, from within the family, the local community and the professional bodies.

*The right to respect for the family and the community*

A central component of 'valuing the individual' is recognising the individual in relation to their family and community, and in challenging oppressive assumptions arising from stereotypical categorisations of both. Hudson (1992:145) argues that a 'fundamental error' of the Cleveland inquiry was in 'subsuming parents in one catch-all category; both the inquiry and much press coverage of child sexual issues has failed to differentiate between mothers and fathers'.

Appreciating power dynamics within families, and recognising the potential for all family members to act as carers are values advocated by CCETSW and reflected in relevant legislation. The lack of power of many mothers and other females within the family structure is to be acknowledged (CCETSW, 1991d:32), with section 8 orders of the Children Act 1989 intending to encourage adults involved to maintain contact where appropriate and possible. Such emphasis values the continuity of significant relationships in the development of good practice. Hudson argues that the Cleveland inquiry placed an almost 'obsessive' emphasis on diagnosis and procedure, and subsequently failed to comment on the ingredients of 'good practice' after a disclosure had been made (Hudson, 1992:140). Good practice accommodates the potential for the wider family networks and support within the community to be used when decisions are to be made with and about the child (CCETSW, 1991d:40; Children Act 1989: section 5(6)). The use of the extended family networks and of the local community coincides with the legislative requirement that only 'positive intervention' is to be made (Children Act 1989: section 1(5)), a requirement which aims to help children and young people identify positive factors about their families wherever possible (CCETSW, 1991d:21, 32). Such legislation is welcome when it is enforced alongside the core value of respect for the cultural and racial context of the family within the community, and acknowledgement of diversity and difference within and between family structure. Practitioners should be prepared to recruit single men and women, gay and lesbian couples and people with disabilities and to assess their ability to parent. Hudson (1992) highlights central concerns of how 'race' and 'homosexuality' are invariably referred to with damaging generalised assumptions. She addresses the detrimental effects this has in the charged moments of the effort to protect the rights of children and parents. Such work argues that the rights of the individual and family should be respected in order to maintain the welfare of the child. Prejudiced value assumptions must be identified and addressed to ensure that the protection of child and adult is maintained.

*Individual right to confidentiality*
The family and community are to be respected for the resources each holds for the development of good enough practice. A central task in maintaining respect is establishing and maintaining clearly defined boundaries between worker and client. In order to maintain such boundaries, value must be placed on the client's right to confidentiality. While the client is entitled to respect, privacy and confidentiality (CCETSW, 1991a:15; 1995:4) the social worker also holds ultimate responsibility for ensuring that information is acted on to give 'protection to those at risk of abuse and exploitation and violence to themselves and others' (CCETSW, 1991a:16). Relevant information must neither be shared around too liberally nor withheld, leaving a vulnerable client in danger. The essential development of good practice suggests that the client and worker clarify the codes of practice around confidentiality (Department of Health, 1991b:11); that the client is informed of the procedures that follow a disclosure, and is consulted during subsequent action. Ensuring that this process takes place requires clearly defined boundaries to exist between worker and client. The often genuine desire to become 'friendly' with the client and to identify shared life experiences can have adverse effects as boundaries are merged. Good supervision will ensure that it is the client's needs which are being identified and met, not the social worker's (Simmonds, 1988).

*Appropriate practice: participation, accountability and*
*accessibility with specific reference to community care*
While the above has addressed the rights of the individual with reference to childcare practice, it must be stressed that such rights are transferable across the range of practice contexts. The case above highlights some of the basic rights of the individual in the development of appropriate practice. Central to this is the recognition of the systemic relationship between the individual within the family, and the family within the community. The emphasis on an accountable, accessible and appropriate practice is a mainstay of the Griffiths Report (Griffiths, 1988), and the Department of Health White Paper (Department of Health, 1989). In this section we address the value placed on self-help and client participation as it pertains to the development of care in the community. At the cost of labouring the same point, while reference is made to work with adults with specific needs (see also Chapter 5), such values are similarly transferable across the range of contexts for social work practice.

The scope to provide appropriate services run in and by the community is the premise for community care legislation which stresses commitment to people being cared for by their family at home, or in a 'homely environment' (Langan, 1990:58). The individual is enabled to achieve greater choice by the encouragement of 'active participation' on the part of both the carer and the cared for (Department of Health, 1989 quoted in Biehal, 1993:443). This is closely aligned with the core values of social work outlined by CCETSW, which stress the need for a commitment to both the strengths and the skills embodied in local communities, and to the right of individuals and families to choose (CCETSW, 1991a:15).

The capacity for individual choice and participation in decision-making has been seen to be undermined through institutional care. Although codes of practice for residential care have invariably echoed core values outlined by CCETSW,[1] studies of powerlessness within institutions have demonstrated how the scope for individual autonomy and choice is undermined by the rituals, regimes and disciplines of the institution (Goffman, 1968; Foucault, 1979; Trevillion, 1992) and by the interaction between different institutions involved in the delivery of care. The postwar decline in popularity of institutional care is clearly depicted by Langan, who refers to a sequence of government reports and White Papers in the 1960s and 1970s which echoed a consensus in favour of community care by many service users (Langan, 1990:60).[2]

The emphasis on community care within the National Health Service and Community Care Act 1990 has stressed the increased scope for practitioners to be accountable to the client and community they serve. Such accountability cannot be achieved, however, by the worker alone: community resources must be made available. Despite the enthusiasm for Care in the Community, its achievements in practice have not been without criticism. For example, the premature closure of hospitals under the mental hospital closure programme has been criticised for not allowing time for due consideration of the availability of alternative resources to meet individual need (Jones, 1989). The tragic events resulting from people returning to the community without due consideration being given to their needs illustrates the severe practical implications when core values, such as respecting and assessing individual need, are ignored (Langan, 1990). The concept of 'dangerousness' referred to earlier returns here, as a specific and immediate danger to the community can result from inadequate support being made available to the vulnerable adult. Damage can also be done to the unsupported carer, often a woman: it is usually women who bear the brunt of care within the family and community (Langan, 1990:58–70). The attraction of promoting individual rights and choices by returning individuals to the community can override the core values of challenging the negative discrimination that is experienced by many carers. It can also undermine the right to protection of those at risk of abuse to themselves and others (CCETSW, 1991a:15–16). With this in mind, due consideration must be given to the potential exploitation of the carer within the private domain, and to the emotional, personal and physical needs of the client.

### Participation and user rights: difference and diversity within the community

The section above which discussed individual rights in relation to childcare practice argued that value judgements should not be made about an individual's capacity to parent or care for a child because of their racial origin, age, sexual orientation or their gender. Similarly, policy and practice interventions aiming to develop Care in the Community must not assume that all users participate and benefit from local provision (Biehal, 1993). Upholding the theoretical proposal that community care 'can be a strategy for upholding the rights of users to be treated as full and equal citizens', Biehal concentrates on the practical application of 'participation' as founded upon 'a commitment to users' rights' (Biehal, 1993:444). The promotion of participation through 'mission statements' is not a guarantee that all users will participate equally in practice. Genuine participation occurs if users have rights to negotiate decisions at every level of decision-making. Referring to her study of the individual contacts between workers in social care and older people, Biehal looked at the way in which 'service users were encouraged to express their own view of their needs' (Biehal, 1993:445). Her study encouraged professionals to consider the ways in which the inequality of power between professionals and service users resulted in definitions of need being made 'on behalf of users rather than in partnership with them' (Biehal, 1993:446).

Stereotypical assumptions are inherent in the decision-making process on behalf of users. These assumptions have been challenged in relation to the concept of working with 'communities of interests', outlined by the Barclay Report (Barclay, 1982:xiii). Preferring to refer to 'social networks which develop around an awareness of oppression' rather than communities of interest, Trevillion recognises the need for the accommodation of diversity and conflict within communities and networks (Trevillion, 1992:83–5). He sees considerable scope in community care legislation, particularly in its potential for promoting self-help and self-advocacy, through which individuals have an opportunity to define their own needs and interests. He refers to the development of organisations such as Body Positive and Positively Women which 'have grown out of a community's discovery of itself and its power' (Trevillion, 1992:85). Such networks of interest arise from the need for individuals to represent themselves, as opposed to being represented by others. This accommodates self-defined differences between individual experiences, and creates opportunities for empowerment where the social worker functions in a partnership which recognises the individual circumstance (Trevillion, 1992:83–97). This interpretation of networks of interests is attractive, as the worker becomes accountable to individual clients' needs within the community, and to the relevant networks of interest.

The value of working in partnership and of maintaining an accountable service, as outlined above, is described by CCETSW in its analysis of disability issues (CCETSW, 1991c). Many disabled people have become increasingly critical of support services offered to them. Social work practice has been criticised for failing to consult the client, making assumptions about individual need from a medical rather than social concept of disability (CCETSW, 1991c:13). In this context, scope for change and improvement exists within the legislative requirements of the NHS and Community Care Act 1990. This stipulates that social worker and client be intricately involved with the assessments of need and management of support services (CCETSW, 1991c:14–15). Such practice, for example user involvement, the encouragement of consumer choice and the maintenance of an accountable, multi-disciplinary service, creates a 'social model' rather than an individual medical model.

The emphasis on self-determination, and on the client-led services which are prevalent within de-institutionalisation and community care legislation, is endorsed by campaigners calling for the 'normalisation' of people with learning difficulties. Williams (1992:142) argues that the aim of such changes is to

> provide ways for people with learning difficulties to integrate into the mainstream of society, to participate and be valued members of society and enjoy the same rights, opportunities and patterns of living as others in society.

Williams identifies the development of self-advocacy groups as providing ways of empowering people, encouraging more equal and cooperative relationship between service users and providers.

The appropriation of power by able-bodied society, with the subsequent devaluation of respect and dignity for the individual with a disability or with a learning difficulty, has perpetuated the dependency of disabled people on the able-bodied community (Oliver, 1991). The publication of a CCETSW-funded guide to community care by and for people with learning difficulties shows how the individual users can challenge such negative discrimination by participating in their own assessment and in the management of their care plan (People First, 1993). However, as argued earlier, respecting the individual must mean that all forms of oppression be considered together. For example, the focus on 'self' in 'self-advocacy' should ensure that services in the community are not developed only within a Eurocentric perspective which at best assumes its accessibility to 'others' and at worst actively excludes 'others'. CCETSW argues that, 'given the historic failure to deliver appropriate personal social services to their community', the new agenda for action will need close scrutiny (CCETSW, 1991c:122). At the same time, CCETSW (1991b:89) recognises racism as a fundamental problem by stating that 'it is possible that many black clients are not convinced that social workers are committed to upholding civil rights or equality for black people'. The 'mission' espoused by the provider (CCETSW, 1991c:20) must therefore challenge discrimination and attempt to remain accessible to the community it serves. The provider must develop a business plan which analyses the external environment from a range of perspectives, which include economic, sociocultural and politico-legal.

This demonstrates the fact that deeds speak more than words. That is to say, the value of empowering and enabling clients of diverse social and cultural backgrounds should not be treated as conveying a slogan. The good intention must be translated into effective practice by actively engaging and applying the principles discussed in this chapter.

### Commitment to social justice and social welfare: from Care in the Community to control by the community

The previous sections addressed core values which place priority on respect for the individual, and referred to the values and strengths of working within the 'community'. Central to the themes covered is the need to challenge negative discrimination. In this section we refer to social work with offenders, drawing on the core values identified above as transferable across the range of practice, while elaborating on the value of expressing a commitment to social justice and social welfare (CCETSW, 1991a:15; 1995:26).

As with all areas of practice, knowledge of the relationship between the individual viewpoint of the practitioner, the requirements of the professional role, and of the overall function of the agency within the system is essential. Knowledge of how basic social work values apply within the criminal justice system is of paramount importance. As Denney (1991:61) suggests:

The approach to probation training rightly points to the fact that lack of basic knowledge can tragically affect the outcome of social work intervention. It can also be argued that a failure to locate racism in organisational structures can have devastating effects on the quality of service delivered to the recipients of probation services.

The Home Office concentration on 'new realist values in probation', where emphasis is placed on the offence committed as opposed to the social history of the offender, challenges the 'therapeutic optimism' of the probation service of the 1960s and 1970s (Willis, 1981). This is further reflected in vague government intentions to separate probation training from social work education (Denney, 1991:61; Home Office, 1995a, 1995b; Nellis, 1996). The more welcomed proposal of discrete training for probation officers alongside an integrated generic social work foundation course provides scope for students to concentrate on the development of shared knowledge, values and skills, making connections between and within the role of probation and other social work disciplines. This emphasis opens up the scope for the caring credo: 'an attitude towards suspects, accused persons and prisoners based on liberal and humanitarian values' to be understood alongside the punishment credo: 'the punitive degradation of offenders' (Lord Scarman, quoted in Rutherford, 1993:viii). Rutherford argues that practitioners at all levels of the criminal justice system play a central role in expressing humane values. While he emphasises the importance of knowledge of the ideologies and values espoused by the practitioner, he also recognises two other ways by which 'the pervasive but often concealed relationship between values and criminal justice' is exerted. These are the formal legislation and the structural arrangements of the criminal justice system (Rutherford, 1993:1–2).

With respect to formal legislation, the Criminal Justice Act 1991, with its 1993 amendments (see also Chapter 6 in this volume for further comment), places emphasis on the punishment credo, acknowledging research which argues that custody is a poor deterrent to further offending (Home Office, 1990) and has little value in enhancing human dignity.[3] The Act attempts to ensure that custody is withheld as a sentence for the minority of serious offenders (section 1(2) (a)), while community-based sentences are promoted for those with less serious offences. Custody is to be imposed by the court to protect the public from serious harm. This attempt to reduce the use of custody for minor offences should be welcomed, since research into the use of custodial sentences suggests that some practices under the auspice of pursuit of social justice have perpetuated, as opposed to challenged, negative discrimination. For example, black people with learning difficulties or mental health problems have been found to be over-represented within institutional provision (Browne, 1990; Francis, 1991: 81–2) and women have been found to be judged according to their conformity to the stereotypical feminine image as well as for their offence (Gelsthorpe, 1989; Cain, 1989). Furthermore, some evidence suggests that miscarriages of justice have occurred when some offenders, who pleaded not guilty, without a pre-sentence report in Crown Court, were sentenced to custody: a disproportionately high number of these were black offenders (NACRO, 1993:5). The damaging use of racist stereotypes and symbols, as opposed to a non-judgmental assessment of the reality of individual behaviour, may reveal more about the 'ideological baggage' of white people than about the families of black people (Pitts, 1993).

The Criminal Justice Act 1991, and 1993 amendments, is the first recognition in statute law of the duty of those administering criminal justice to avoid discrimination (Home Office and NACRO, 1992). Section 95 of the 1991 Act insists that those administering criminal justice should 'avoid discrimination against persons on the ground of race or sex or any other improper ground' (Criminal Justice Act 1991: section 95).

While these developments are welcomed, conflicts arise between differing values of some of the CCETSW requirements and those proposed by the Home Office within legislative reform. For example, the government's exploration of the use of private companies or trusts in the delivery of services raises concern as to how CCETSW's demand for a non-oppressive, anti-racist and anti-sexist service will be maintained in the demand/profit-led ethos (Denney, 1991:60). Similarly, the emphasis on the 'punishment credo' is extended as the concept of punishment within the community is developed (Criminal Justice Act 1991: sections 6, 10). This emphasis on the punishment credo within the legislation explained above raises concern about the long-term effects of the limited scope for preventative and flexible responses to offending behaviour within local communities.

This brings us to Rutherford's second concern: where he asks for an analysis of values within the structural arrangements of the criminal justice system. Whatever the legislative framework, the individual practitioner's values can never be divorced from the reality of local and specific experience. For example, despite the creation of national standards as an attempt to maintain quality assurance across local variations, and to ensure that the sentence reflects the seriousness of the offence (the Proportionality Principle, Criminal Justice Act 1991: sections 18(2), 6(1), (1(2)) the interpretation of sentencing guidelines could, if used wrongly, with too little account taken of personal mitigation and other contributing items, undermine that intent. NACRO (1993:12) warns that there is a possibility that this could 'escalate sentencing, with serious cost implications', and undermine much progressive community-based work.

As practitioners are working with different magistrates, in different services and with diverse community resources, it is important that there ought to be some common and uniform service delivery without challenging regional 'individuality'. The need to maintain the respect for the individual while responding to the strengths and skills of different local communities will be pertinent to working with offenders. Central to the debates around the changes in recent legislation and structural arrangements to social work with offenders is the attempt to maintain core values while responding to the increasing demand for an accountable service within often poorly resourced and overstretched communities. The centre stage of any good social work practice, including the supervision of offenders, still consists of the same values: a commitment to the dignity of all individuals irrespective of their specific background and location; respect for privacy and confidentiality; respect for the rights of clients and their families to know the options, the reason for intervention and their involvement in shaping, as far as is possible, their future. This means recognising, as well as promoting, the strengths and skills to be found in local communities. *In toto*, the core aim of any social work practitioner should be to strive towards establishing working 'partnerships' and empowering participants to exercise their rights and enable them to make choices. Even in cases where choice may appear to be limited, as for example in administering penal sanctions, at every stage of the social and legal relationships that take place the defendant, or victim or their families have rights and choices which they should be made aware of and encouraged to exercise. For example, notwithstanding the problematic nature of 'consent' in the administration of community service orders (Vass, 1984) the defendant is entitled to receive clear guidelines and options prior to being invited to consent. Consent can be his or her right to accept or reject punishment but should not be denied or used as a means by which the defendant is coerced into submission for fear that some other more painful punishment would be in the offing.

The practitioner has the responsibility to communicate clearly with clients, informing them of these rights and choices. This is reflected in all areas of practice, and its importance cannot be underestimated. While external resources diminish, increasing emphasis is placed on the importance of the practitioner as a resource. Responsibility is placed on the individual to deliver a non-oppressive and accountable service. The recent literature on 'empowerment' stresses this theme within social work theory and practice.

It is with this in mind that we conclude by looking at the use of self as the location for the development of competent practice.

## Conclusion

> The starting point of critical elaboration is the consciousness of what one really is, and is knowing thyself as a product of the historical process to date which has deposited in you an infinity of traces, without leaving an inventory. (Gramsci, 1971:324)

The above quotation asks that priority be placed on knowledge of self, located within and determined by historical events, privileged with the scope to create change. The complexities of such emphasis are becoming more apparent as the professional use of self is incorporated into the analysis of anti-discriminatory practice. In short, the core values of social work can be stated and promoted as this chapter has attempted to do, but some values have no significance or meaning unless they are internalised. The individual social worker must believe in those values and apply them in practice.

An increasing body of literature is addressing the need to use good supervision as a mechanism for exposing concerns around difference between self and other (Yelloly, 1993). The use of self in the professional's capacity to stand back and take a wider, non-prejudicial view is being explored and projected as a means of developing practice which challenges negative discrimination (Loughlin, 1992; Frosh, 1987; Yelloly, 1993). For example, the use of psychodynamic theories, informed by political awareness of structural inequalities, provides a context within which prejudice can be localised and individualised (Payne, 1992). The processes of transference and counter-transference can reveal the distinction between the needs of the client and the needs of the worker (Brown and Pearce, 1992:163). Good supervision helps to identify 'difference' as it arises in practice, enabling workers to ensure that 'their own values and prejudices do not detract from their professional objectivity' (Department of Health and Social Security, 1988:10).

Such processes can ensure that a special commitment to anti-discriminatory practice is made and that mechanisms develop for monitoring one's own and others' difficulties in this area in efforts to develop a more appropriate practice (CCETSW, 1991a, 1991b, 1991c, 1991d, 1995).

The challenge for social work is to deliver an appropriate non-oppressive practice. This means making constructive accommodation of the lessons from the past while adhering to a set of core values without colluding with popular attempts, from a range of political perspectives, to undermine social work's professional development.

## Notes

1. For example the rights of residents to achieve their potential capacity at a physical, intellectual, emotional and social level; their rights to dignity, autonomy and individuality; and their rights to have their qualities, experiences and talents respected.

2. Accepting the ideological preference for community care in theory is different from accepting its implementation in practice. Resource allocation to local authorities has invariably failed to meet the demands placed upon the community, where often poorly trained staff struggle to meet the basic needs of their client group.

3. The Criminal Justice Act's main theme of expanding community penalties and establishing prison as a last resort run counter to the current expansion of prison regimes, and the claim by Mr Michael Howard, the Home Secretary, that 'prison works' (see Vass, 1996).

## References

Ahmed, S., Cheetham, J. and Small, J. (1986) *Social Work with Black Children and their Families*. London: Batsford in association with British Agencies for Adoption and Fostering.

Bailey, R. and Brake, M. (1975) *Radical Social Work*. London: Arnold.

Barclay, P.M. (1982) *Social Workers: Their Roles and Tasks*. London: National Institute of Social Work/Bedford Square Press (Barclay Report).

Beistek, F.P. (1965) *The Casework Relationship*. London: Allen & Unwin.

Beveridge, W. (1942) *Social Insurance and Allied Services* (Cmd 6404). London: HMSO.

Biehal, N. (1993) 'Changing practice: participation, rights and community care', *British Journal of Social Work*, 23(5): 443–58.

Blackburn, C. (1991) *Poverty and Health: Working with Families*. Milton Keynes: Open University Press.

Booth, General William (1890) 'In darkest England and the way out', in K. Woodroofe (1962) *From Charity to Social Work in England and the United States*. London: Routledge & Kegan Paul. pp. 18–20.

Brown, H.C. (1992) 'Lesbians, the state, and social work practice', in M. Langan and L. Day (eds), *Women, Oppression and Social Work*. London: Routledge. pp. 201–19.

Brown, H.C. and Pearce, J.J. (1992) 'Good practice in the face of anxiety: social work with girls and young women', *Journal of Social Work Practice*, 6(2): 159–65.

Browne, D. (1990) *Black People, Mental Health and the Courts*. London: National Association for the Care and Resettlement of Offenders.

Cain, M. (1989) *Growing Up Good – Policing the Behaviour of Girls in Europe*. London: Sage.

Campbell, B. (1993) *Goliath: Britain's Dangerous Places*. London: Methuen.

Carter, P., Jeffs, T. and Smith, M. (1992) *Changing Social Work and Welfare*. Milton Keynes: Open University Press.

CCETSW (1991a) *DipSW: Rules and Requirements for the Diploma in Social Work* (Paper 30), 2nd edn. London: Central Council for Education and Training in Social Work.

CCETSW (1991b) *CCETSW Study 8: One Small Step towards Racial Justice: the Teaching of Anti-racism in Diploma in Social Work Programmes*. London: Central Council for Education and Training in Social Work.

CCETSW (1991c) *CCETSW Study 9: Disability Issues – Developing Anti-Discriminatory Practice*. London: Central Council for Education and Training in Social Work.

CCETSW (1991d) *The Teaching of Child Care in the Diploma in Social Work*. London: Central Council for Education and Training in Social Work.

CCETSW (1995) *DipSW: Rules and Requirements for the Diploma in Social Work* (Paper 30), revised edn. London: Central Council for Education and Training in Social Work.

Cheetham, J. (ed.) (1981) *Social Work and Ethnicity*. London: Allen & Unwin.

Clark, C.L. and Asquith, S. (1985) *Social Work and Social Philosophy*. London: Routledge & Kegan Paul.

Conn, J. and Turner, A. (1990) 'Working with women in families', in R. Perlberg and A. Miller (eds), *Gender and Power in Families*. London: Routledge. pp. 175–91.

Cypher, J. (1975) 'Social reform and the social work profession: what hope for a rapprochement', in H. Jones (ed.), *Towards a New Social Work*. London: Routledge & Kegan Paul. pp. 4–25.

Davies, M. (1985) *The Essential Social Worker: A Guide to Positive Practice*. Aldershot: Gower.

Denney, D. (1991) 'Anti-racism, probation training and the criminal justice system', in CCETSW, *One Small Step towards Racial Justice: the Teaching of Anti-racism in Diploma in Social Work Programmes*. London: Central Council for Education and Training in Social Work. pp. 58–80.

Department of Health (1989) *Caring for People: Community Care in the Next Decade and Beyond*. London: HMSO.

Department of Health (1991a) *Child Abuse. A Study of Inquiry Reports 1980–1989*. London: HMSO.

Department of Health (1991b) *Protecting Children: A Guide for Social Workers Undertaking a Comprehensive Assessment*. London: HMSO.

Department of Health and Social Security (1988) *Report of the Inquiry into Child Abuse in Cleveland 1987: Short Version Extracted from the Complete Text*. London: HMSO.

Dominelli, L. (1988) *Anti-Racist Social Work*. London: Macmillan.

Dominelli, L. and McLeod, E. (1989) *Feminist Social Work*. London: Macmillan.

Foucault, M. (1979) *Discipline and Punish: the Birth of the Prison*. Harmondsworth: Penguin.

Foucault, M. (1991) 'Governmentality', in G. Burchell, C. Gordon and P. Miller, *The Foucault Effect: Studies in Governmentality*. Hemel Hempstead: Harvester Wheatsheaf. pp. 87–104.

Francis, E. (1991) 'Mental health, antiracism and social work training', in CCETSW, *One Small Step towards Racial Justice: the Teaching of Anti-racism in Diploma in Social Work Programmes* London: Central Council for Education and Training in Social Work. pp. 81–95.

Frosh, S. (1987) *The Politics of Psychoanalysis*. London: Macmillan.

Gelsthorpe, L. (1989) *Sexism and the Female Offender* (Cambridge Studies in Criminology). Aldershot: Gower.

Gilroy, P. (1987) *There Ain't No Black in the Union Jack*. London: Hutchinson.

Glendinning, C. and Millar, J. (eds) (1992) *Women and Poverty in Britain: the 1990s*. Hemel Hempstead: Harvester Wheatsheaf.

Goffman, E. (1968) *Asylums: Essays on the Social Situation of Mental Patients and Other Inmates*. Harmondsworth: Penguin.

Gramsci, A. (1971) 'The study of philosophy', in *Selections from Prison Notebooks*. London: Lawrence & Wishart. pp. 323–77.

Griffiths, R. (1988) *Community Care: Agenda for Action*. London: HMSO.

Hardy, J. (1981) *Values in Social Policy: Nine Contradictions*. London: Routledge & Kegan Paul.

Harker, A. (1992) 'Trust in the future: an examination of the changing nature of charitable trusts', in P. Carter, T. Jeffs and M.K. Smith (eds), *Changing Social Work and Welfare*. Milton Keynes: Open University Press.

Home Office (1990) *Crime, Justice and Protecting the Public* (CM 965. London: HMSO.

Home Office (1991) *Working Together under the Children Act 1989*. London: HMSO.

Home Office (1995a) *Review of Probation Officer Recruitment and Qualifying Training. Discussion Paper by the Home Office*. London: Home Office.

Home Office (1995b) *Review of Probation Officer Recruitment and Qualifying Training. Decision Paper by the Home Office*. London: Home Office (mimeo).

Home Office and National Association for the Care and Resettlement of Offenders [NACRO] (1992) *The Criminal Justice Act 1991: A Quick Reference Guide for the Probation Service*. London: HMSO.

Hudson, A. (1992) 'The child sexual abuse "industry" and gender relations in social work', in M. Langan and L. Day (eds), *Women, Oppression and Social Work: Issues in Anti-Discriminatory Practice*. London: Routledge. pp. 129–48.

Jones, K. (1989) 'Community care: old problems and new answers', in P. Carter, T. Jeffs and M. Smith (eds), *Social Work and Social Welfare Yearbook 1*. Milton Keynes: Open University Press. pp. 112–13.

Langan, M. (1990) 'Community care in the 1990s: the community care White Paper: Caring for People', *Critical Social Policy*, 29: 58–70.

Langan, M. and Day, L. (eds) (1992) *Women, Oppression and Social Work: Issues in Anti-Discriminatory Practice*. London: Routledge.

Langan, M. and Lee, P. (1989) *Radical Social Work Today*. London: Unwin Hyman.

London Borough of Brent (1985) *A Child in Trust: Report on the Death of Jasmine Beckford*. London: London Borough of Brent.

Loughlin, B. (1992) 'Supervision in the face of no cure – working on the boundary', *Journal of Social Work Practice*, 6(2): 111–16.

Lukacs, G. (1971) *History and Class Consciousness: Studies in Marxist Dialectics*. London: Merlin Press.

Macdonald, S. (1991) *All Equal under the Act? A Practical Guide to the Children Act 1989 for Social Workers*. Manchester: Race Equality Unit, Manchester/Pankhurst Press. pp. 88–9.

Mannheim, K. (1948) *Ideology and Utopia*. London: Routledge.

Maslow, A. (1970) *Motivation and Personality*, 2nd edn. New York: Harper & Row.

Meikle, J. (1994) 'Patten basics guide to go to all homes', *Guardian*, 8 January.

Mercer, K. (1990) 'Welcome to the jungle: identity and diversity in postmodern politics', in J. Rutherford (ed.), *Identity. Community, Culture, Difference.* London: Lawrence & Wishart. pp. 43–71.

Moore, S. (1993) 'Not a single issue', *Guardian*, 16 July.

National Association for the Care and Resettlement of Offenders [NACRO] (1993) *Juveniles Remanded in Custody* (NACRO Briefing Paper). London: NACRO.

Nellis, M. (1996) 'Probation training: the links with social work', in T. May and A.A. Vass (eds), *Working with Offenders: Issues, Contexts and Outcomes.* London: Sage. pp. 7–30.

Oliver, M. (1990) *The Politics of Disablement* London: Macmillan.

Oliver, M. (1991) *Social Work: Disabled People and Disabling Environments.* London: Jessica Kingsley.

Page, R. (1992) 'Empowerment, oppression and beyond: a coherent strategy? A reply to Ward and Mullender', *Critical Social Policy*, 35: 89–92.

Payne, M. (1991) *Modern Social Work Theory: a Critical Introduction.* London: Macmillan.

Payne, M. (1992) 'Psychodynamic theory within the politics of social work theory', *Journal of Social Work Practice*, 6(2): 141–9.

Peacock, G. and Collins, S. (1989) *Social Work and Received Ideas.* London: Routledge.

Pearson, G. (1983) *Hooligan: A History of Respectable Fears.* London: Macmillan.

Pearson, G., Treseder, J. and Yelloly, M. (eds) (1988) *Social Work and the Legacy of Freud: Psychoanalysis and its Uses.* London: Macmillan.

People First (1993) *'Oi! It's My Assessment' All You Have Ever Wanted to Know about Community Care.* London: People First.

Pitts, J. (1993) 'Thereotyping: anti-racism, criminology and black young people', in D. Cooke and B. Hudson (eds), *Racism and Criminology.* London: Sage. pp. 96–117.

Probyn, E. (1993) *Sexing the Self: Gendered Positions in Cultural Studies.* London: Routledge. pp. 1–6.

Rogers, C.R. (1951) *Client Centre Therapy: Its Current Practice Implications and Theory.* London: Constable.

Rogers, C.R. (1961) *On Becoming a Person: a Therapist's View of Psychotherapy.* London: Constable.

Rowbotham, S., Segal, L. and Wainwright, H. (1979) *Beyond the Fragments: Feminism and the Making of Socialism.* London: Merlin Press.

Rutherford, A. (1993) *Criminal Justice and the Pursuit of Decency.* Oxford: Oxford University Press.

Seidler, V.J. (1991) *Recreating Sexual Politics.* London: Routledge.

Shardlow, S. (ed.) (1989) *The Values of Change in Social Work.* London and New York: Tavistock/Routledge.

Simmonds, J. (1988) 'Thinking about feelings in group care', in G. Pearson, J. Treseder and M. Yelloly (eds), *Social Work and the Legacy of Freud: Psychoanalysis and its Uses.* London: Macmillan. pp. 202–15.

Spelman, E.V. (1988) *Inessential Woman: Problems of Exclusion in Feminist Thought.* London: The Women's Press.

Timms, N. and Timms, R. (1977) *Perspectives in Social Work.* London: Routledge & Kegan Paul.

Trevillion, S. (1992) *Caring in the Community: A Network Approach to Community Partnership.* Harlow: Longman.

Vass, A.A. (1984) *Sentenced to Labour: Close Encounters with a Prison Substitute.* St Ives: Venus Academica.

Vass, A.A. (1986) *AIDS: a Plague in Us: a Social Perspective. The Condition and its Social Consequences.* St Ives: Venus Academica.

Vass, A.A. (1996) 'Community penalties: the politics of punishment', in T. May and A.A. Vass (eds), *Working with Offenders: Issues, Contexts and Outcomes.* London: Sage. pp. 157–84.

Ward, D. and Mullender, A. (1991) 'Empowerment and oppression: an indissoluble pairing for contemporary social work', *Critical Social Policy*, 32: 21–30.

White, R., Carr, P. and Lowe, N. (1990) *A Guide to the Children Act 1989.* London: Butterworth.

Williams, F. (1992) 'Women with learning difficulties are women too', in M. Langan and L. Day (eds), *Women, Oppression and Social Work: Issues in Anti-discriminatory Practice.* London: Routledge. pp. 149–68.

Willis, C. (1981) 'Effective criminal supervision – towards new standards and goals'. Lecture to the National Association of Probation Officers Branch Day Conference, Darlington.

Woodroofe, K. (1962) *From Charity to Social Work in England and the United States.* London: Routledge & Kegan Paul.

Yelloly, M. (1993) 'The dynamics of difference: poverty and wealth', *Journal of Social Work Practice*, 7(1): 5–15.

# 3

# The Core Skills of Social Work

In the wake of the Children Act 1989, the Criminal Justice Act 1991 and the National Health Service and Community Care Act 1990 and the introduction of the new Diploma in Social Work (CCETSW, 1995), the profession is once again re-examining itself. Part of this re-examination includes attempts at redefinition of skills. The Barclay Report (1982) defined these as 'skills in human relationships, skills in analysis . . . and skills in effectiveness'. These skills require fresh consideration, but whether new skills are required, or whether these are in effect any different from past skills is a matter for debate.

In the context of care management, for example, is it just the acquiring of new skills which is being demanded or is a different kind of social worker needed (Orme and Glastonbury, 1993)? What is different about working in partnership with users currently and what if anything remains the same? What are necessary skills in developing an empowering practice?

Essentially this chapter will address the question of core skills: what they are, why they are considered necessary and how they are acquired and implemented. Skills development can be seen as a bridge between exploring values, acquiring knowledge and translating these into positive service provision. Without knowledge (e.g. social work theory, research findings, legislation) and without an understanding of how values (e.g. of worker, client, agency, society) affect individual situations, skills remain undefined and vague. 'S/he communicates well', 's/he is good with people', and so on. Operationalising that knowledge and understanding is the bedrock to developing competent practice.

CCETSW Paper 30 (CCETSW, 1991, 1995) identifies five broad categories which incorporate necessary skills. Cognitive skills are identified as the ability to analyse and apply knowledge to practice. Interpersonal skills cover a wide and complex range, for example understanding of self, self in relation to other, locating and working with complicated feelings and situations. Clear communication, and working in partnership are also grouped in this section. Decision-making, administrative skills and the ability to use resources effectively are grouped separately. There is clearly a relationship between each of these categories, and an overlap in the skills used in each.

These have now been superseded by six core competences as part of the rewriting of Paper 30 (see CCETSW, 1995). These competences refer to: communicating and engaging, promoting and enabling; assessing and planning; interviewing and providing services, and working in organisations.

It is however important to acknowledge the fundamental significance of many of the core skills identified in this chapter. They reflect and at the same time complement CCETSW's requirements. In our view they will remain essential components of competent practice in any organisational context and in departmental reorganisations.

Each of the following sections will address these necessary skills underpinning sound practice. Each will consider what they are, how they are acquired and the meaning of their use in current practice. In the context of the continual reorganisation of personal social services these meanings may at times alter in emphasis. With changes of role and job description there may be more emphasis in some roles on, for example, administrative skills than interpersonal skills. However, without the latter the former cannot happen and it is with this in mind that the following sections seek to provide a broadly based look at the developments of significant skills for service provision, working in 'partnership with members of the community' and 'collaborating with colleagues and workers in other organisations' (CCETSW, 1991, 1995).

### Cognitive skills

Developing analytic skills, a capacity to evaluate, using research findings effectively, and applying this knowledge and understanding to practice are the cornerstones to developing competence in this area. We need to think further about the meaning of these phrases.

The importance of research to social work practice and the active use of research to inform the work is as comparatively recent as the development of social work itself following the publication of the Seebohm Report (1968). Broadly it could be placed in three main categories:

1. Research following some tragedy or traumatic event, which includes inquiry reports (Department of Health, 1991b);
2. Empirical research addressing the experiences of, for example, managers, workers and users of services (Cleaver and Freeman, 1994; Gibbons, 1993), or addressing the administration of service

provision, the enforcement of community service orders and the effectiveness of community penalties (McIvor, 1992; Raynor, 1988; Vass, 1984, 1990);

3.  Statistical research addressing such concerns as the operation of child protection registers (Little and Gibbons, 1993), provision of care in the community (Department of Health, 1989a, 1990).

Clearly, research knowledge has different functions but essentially it conveys a pattern which can then contribute to outcomes (Department of Health, 1991c). Each of the above three areas has a relevance to planning of policy and organisation of services to carry out that policy. Recommendations from the *Study of Inquiry Reports* (Department of Health, 1991b) for example address the agency context, issues for management and the management of individual cases. At another level, research findings on the supervision of offenders in the community have led to amendments in penal policy, and the introduction of national standards in an effort to reduce diversity, improve service delivery and instruct as well as enable social workers and probation officers in the field to carry out their tasks in a non-discriminatory manner (Home Office et al., 1995). Each of these sections contains recommendations and proposals. While these themselves will be mediated in individual contexts, adapting relevant essentials could give a general direction to providing services of a similar quality nationwide.

Empirical research, while geographically specific, can at least stimulate thinking about the congruence between users' experiences and service provision. At most it can provide the framework of a particular service, as well as the basis for creating a dialogue between users and providers/policy-makers. It can also offer a sense of the individual experience of workers, managers or users which can be individually confirming or challenging and can collectively contribute to considering for example training packages and consultancy/supervision issues.

Statistical information is particularly useful in planning services, organising budgets and developing policy. Predictive figures in relation to child protection registers can determine the size of team to provide direct work, determine consideration of residential and fostering provision and possible budgetary allocation for training in this area of work. They might also lead to a reconsideration of localised criteria for placement on the register or reconsideration of the way in which separate categories are used and viewed.

This area of research is especially important for practitioners in terms of what can be learnt from previous actions in practice. It has also been enshrined in legislation. For example, the paramountcy principle in the Children Act 1989 could in part be directly attributed to the importance of maintaining focus on the child, a focus which became lost in the Jasmine Beckford and Tyra Henry cases with tragic consequences (Department of Health, 1991b). There is a link between reading and understanding research or research-based material, translating this into organisational ideas of ideas for practice and the development of analytic skills. None of these areas excludes any of the others or exists in isolation; they are interlinked, overlap, and if brought together should provide a complementary experience of service delivery. Certainly the degree of analysis will vary according to context, and different roles will dictate different bases for the development of analytic skills. Again these may not be completely separate. An analysis of need in a practical situation may not exclude the analysis of the emotional context of that situation at a different time. Knowing that both may be necessary, which takes priority, and at what point, is an analytic process in itself, whatever the role of the worker and whatever the context. The spectrum of analytic skills therefore is wide; a court report offering an in-depth analysis of a child in context at one end of the continuum and a decision about whether to physically touch a child in a tantrum in a residential setting appear both different and connected. Deciding how to help an older person bathe in a residential context is different again, and the differences are often reflected by the organisation in terms of status and expenditure. They can be seen to be connected, however, in relation to the application of a simple or more complex analysis, according to context and role, which in turn leads to sensitive and appropriate practice.

The continuum of analysis happens from the point of referral onwards, and will involve staff who have very different roles in the organisation. The context of this chapter indicates an emphasis on social work skills after the initial referral, which may involve basic advice/information-giving or provision of direct services. Initial skills include some kind of analysis, such as helping the inquirer to clarify the nature of the referral, if necessary. If the referral involves a third party, the status and confidentiality of the information needs to be established; similarly the level of urgency and preferred solution (if any). Differences of language, culture and any specific needs also need to be established as part of the initial analysis regarding the referral, its status, possible allocation, and advice regarding the second stage, which will continue the process of assessment in greater depth. (As this is an extremely important area of practice it will be considered separately later in the chapter.)

Analysis and evaluation are not separate skills. There is an overlap as both are part of a continuum, which aims at imputing meaning to information gathered or received. The notion both of analysis and of evaluation form part of a dynamic process of work from referral to closure. Both need to be consistently present as part of the interaction of worker and client, and clarifying this process is an essential ingredient of working in partnership with users. This is in relation to direct service provision. Evaluation also varies according to role and the context of the work. The skills a team manager employs to evaluate the service will reflect the needs of the agency, the needs of the workers, and the needs of the aspect of the service for which they are responsible. For example, the evaluative skills of a front-line manager responsible for a system of care management would need to include collating information from appropriate monitoring systems, allocation of budgets, analysis of workload and work being undertaken, team developments and evaluating the process of change and its impact on workers and services.

The 1990 government reforms to health and social services created a new context for community teams (Department of Health, 1989a, 1989b, 1990). A quasi-market was established, and social services departments established the principle of the statutory authority as the assessor or purchaser. Providers were independent services, and/ or provider sections of the statutory authority.

Evaluation will differ according to whether the statutory service is deemed to be a purchaser or a provider. For a social worker in a purchasing role, part of an evaluation of client need will be of the services offered to meet that need. As providers, workers will be considering, for example, the quality of care provided and the numbers of requests for specific aspects of care. So again there is a continuum of assessment skills which include developing, monitoring and evaluative systems that affect policy and practice.

The following questions may be helpful in identifying the use of cognitive skills by the worker:

- What do I know about the case? What information is available? Who referred? For what purpose?
- What appears to be the core problem, and the associate problems that I need to focus on?
- What are the facts as opposed to impressions?
- Have I a value position on the matter? That is, have I a particular perspective which I can use to analyse the issue without discriminating against the user's rights and choices?
- What is my analysis of the information I have?
- On what do I base this analysis?

- Is there other information I need to have in order to evaluate? If so, from what source (policy, legislation, research, etc.)?
- What can I learn from any similar situations which may have been recorded?
- How might this affect what I now do, and is this appropriate in this situation?
- Have I clarified what I am doing, and for what reasons, sufficiently for myself, for the client, for the agency, for any relevant external body?

**Administrative skills**

Competent administration at all levels must underpin the social work task. Although some functions are carried out by administrators or managerial staff, social workers still need to be able to maintain an overview of the necessary tasks in relation to their own workload, and the way in which these tasks may need to accommodate other aspects of the service. Organising and prioritising individual workloads is clearly essential, both for the competent provision of service and for the sanity of the worker. This prioritisation may also need to accommodate resource availability and other workers' priorities. So administering individual workloads and understanding the systems of which these are a part interact to enable the worker to organise and plan work successfully, competently and in accordance with agency policy and procedure.

One aspect of the administrative task needs to be explored in detail here as it encompasses so much that is important in the social work role. This is record-keeping and report-writing. Again these will vary according to role, from a brief statement in a service user's file to a complex court report in a child protection case, or a pre-sentence report in a criminal case. The proper presentation of accurate information, whatever the context, is of paramount importance for the well-being of the client.

*Record-keeping and report-writing*

These are essential aspects of the social work task. Yet somehow the how, what and why questions that students and practitioners ask in relation to these aspects are rarely comprehensively responded to in the literature (Ford and Jones, 1987). In order to do so one perhaps needs to be clear about some of the blocks to effective writing skills which social workers may commonly encounter. Boredom or uninterest in the task may produce a reluctance to put pen to paper. Self-consciousness about spelling, diction or grammar may be a feature, lying within the broader concern about producing a public record of what is experienced in the initial stages, as a private activity between social worker and user. Workers may see themselves as lacking skills in expressing what they truly experience. Recording may be sidelined in relation to what is perceived as more urgent and real work with clients. Fear of writing too much or too little may be compounded by insufficient administrative resources or lack of agency guidelines about the written tasks. Equally, the guidelines may be unclear or not relevant. There may be unresolved issues around the ethics of record-keeping (BASW, 1983) and confusion about how to separate facts from opinions and how to distinguish the important from the trivial in records and reports. Caught between a combination of such influences the worker may become confused, feel de-skilled and need to be persuaded that the written aspects of the work serve a purpose in relation to competent practice.

In so far as commentators on the profession have addressed issues of competence in relation to records, the inquiry into the death of Shirley Woodcock in 1984 (Department of Health, 1991b) noted that they should provide the following:

- *factual* accounts of significant actions and decisions taken by the social worker, probation officer or client;
- relevant details of current features of a case via brief three-to-six-monthly reviews;
- cumulatively, a historical account which informs the process of planning;
- a reference point for others to act on in the absence of the allocated worker;
- evidence for court proceedings, especially in the form of reports or affidavits;
- a record for the agency of the worker's performance of statutory functions or execution of agreed policy;
- material for research, review, evaluation, learning and teaching purposes;
- an indication of shortfalls and gaps in services;
- continuity between workers handing over a case;
- improved inter-agency cooperation and information sharing;
- *importantly* facilitation of client participation if records are shared and jointly agreed or provision of a record of involvement which may aid the client in understanding their history.

*Clients' access to what is written about them*
Over the last decade changes in the law and a growing research base have confirmed the need for users of services to have access to

information held about them by professional bodies. The Access to Personal Files Act 1989 and the Access to Health Records Act 1991 give people rights to see manual records concerning them, and the Data Protection Act 1984 accords similar rights with regard to computer-held information.

Doel and Lawson (1986) and Ovretveit (1986) confirm that social workers unused to giving clients access to their records express the following reasons for non-disclosure:

- Clients may be adversely affected by disclosure.
- Workers may be adversely affected, particularly if clients challenge the veracity of their records in court.
- Third parties resist disclosure of their materials.
- Sharing records creates an additional burden of work.
- Disclosure involves establishing a relationship of trust over time, which is not possible with new clients.
- There is a lack of agency guidelines on how or what information should be shared.
- Clients are not interested in access to information.
- Confidential judgements need to be protected.

What the research also establishes is that apart from the reasons which have some form of legal backing, social workers also feel reluctant to share with their clients the judgements they reach about eligibility for services or indeed their diagnostic judgements in non-statutory cases which do not require confidentiality in the same way but form a collection of 'clinical musings'. Overall then, the difficulties are based on a constellation of personal fears, professional concerns and lack of agency guidelines or instructions. This lack of openness goes contrary to both legislative requirements and the values of social work in empowering clients (see Chapter 2 on values). As well as violating legal and value requirements, such practice also leads to poor standards in service provision. The same research studies find a number of advantages in pursuing a policy and practice of access:

- Clients can challenge and amend statements which somehow misrepresent them or are inaccurate.
- Partnership becomes a more explicit possibility where clients have some say in what is recorded about them.
- It enables workers to recognise and attempt to fill the gaps which may exist between what they say about empowerment of the client and what they do about it. Honesty, openness and trust are tested out pragmatically.

- Other agencies and professions which are less willing than social work to disclose information become more conscious about disclosure and the legal framework which supports it.
- Writing factually in a language the client understands is developed over time as a specific skill, and re-emphasises the need to avoid jargon.
- Negotiating skills are sharpened in dialogue with clients about the content of records and reports.

*Some guidelines for competent practice*

Social workers should aim to keep records and reports concise, as objective as possible, and readable. Sources need to be stated, and where information is not supported by evidence, facts must be distinguished from conjecture. Having said this, perhaps it is worth indicating where extensive note-keeping may be necessary:

- when statutory proceedings are under way to provide evidence in court;
- monitoring contact between parents and children where quality of interaction is being assessed;
- in relation to reports of non-accidental injury to children, including the details of investigation and assessment, identifying how local and national guidelines for interventions in such cases have been followed;
- where there are complex financial arrangements;
- when complaints have been made by clients about workers, including residential carers;
- when clients are seeking to challenge a refusal of service.

While this is not an exhaustive list, it works along the principle that only a minority of cases and situations require detailed records to be kept and that a balance needs to be struck between too much detail for everyday use and too little detail for evidential purposes. Judgement also needs to be exercised in creating records and reports which meet their purpose and make sense to the reader, for example in separating fact from opinion. Similarly, avoid technical language which mystifies rather than clarifies the writer's view (using words such as sociopathic, labelling, subculture, sibling, enuretic, phobic, insight, feedback) and which may appear meaningful to the social worker, but in fact may diminish the quality of communication between the writer and the readership. Value judgements which give the appearance of professional assessments do so as well, as in this example:

Mrs X is a complex and rather neurotic woman who, not having been adequately parented herself, is now unable to provide for her family. She dresses inappropriately and the house is messy and smells.

This type of clinical musing, with no evidence by way of observed behaviour, does leave the reader wondering whether Mrs X herself would have a view similar to that of the worker. Indeed, the 'metaphor' leaves much to the imagination – what exactly does it refer to, and how much relevance does it have to understanding the user's problems and needs? The following questions may be worth asking when developing the skills for appraisal of a written account:

- Is it relevant to its purpose?
- Is it reliable? Can others vouch for its authenticity? If not, do I make this lack of evidence clear?
- Is it factually accurate?
- Is it hearsay? Especially within a legal context one needs to guard against acting in a manner contrary to the rules of evidence.
- Is it balanced, and non-discriminatory? For example, does it avoid negative stereotypes or recognise and validate client strengths?
- Has it been shared where possible with the client, and has the client been given relevant information about his/her rights?
- Have the client's views about the content of the written account been officially recorded?

Written accounts are increasingly computerised, so a working knowledge of information technology is rapidly becoming an essential administrative skill in the social work task. This is of developing importance for individual workloads and also opens up opportunities to use information stored elsewhere in the department. This growing use of technology also links with the use of research findings and current literature, making this information more immediately accessible and therefore more immediately part of social work practice. While sometimes seen in isolation, competent administrative skills can have far-reaching positive and negative effects in service development, delivery and outcome.

### Interpersonal skills

Interpersonal skills underpin social work practice at all levels throughout the period of user contact. An ability to communicate verbally, non-verbally and in writing is essential (Barclay, 1982; CCETSW, 1991, 1995). Communicating effectively – that is to say, in a way that can be easily understood by others whatever their situation and however different from the worker's – is difficult enough in itself. For this communication to be both meaningful and useful, to be able to be acted on, to make a difference, the response to it also needs to be heard, understood in all its simplicity and complexity, and again used actively. This notion of a developing conversation then builds the user/worker relationship around the task or situation. It creates a working partnership or a relationship where roles are clearly defined and understood. The responsibility for maintaining the boundaries of these relationships lies clearly with the worker (Ahmad, 1990).

There are key elements to interpersonal relationships between social worker and user. The way in which these elements are deployed and with what emphasis will vary according to the individual situation.

### Understanding of self/self-awareness

It may be controversial to place this at the top of the list. However, without that awareness the other elements are liable to distortion. The relationship may founder altogether or become tangled in an unhelpful way, thus obscuring both roles and task. Self-awareness does not only mean an awareness of the meaning of personal history for the worker, and how that personal history may at times interact with a user's personal history, with an ensuing impact on the work. It also implies an understanding of the impact of difference in the working relationship, and how such difference may affect both process and outcome (Conn and Turner, 1990). A worker may choose a particular theoretical model to explore this further or may do so through, for instance, training in the workplace, but the importance of making any difference overt, especially in the context of differing power relationships according to role, has been sub-stantiated in a range of texts (Ahmad, 1990; Kareem and Littlewood, 1992; Langan and Day, 1992). This will be developed in a wider sense later. Here we are concerned with the individual situation and how unacknowledged difference will in some way impact detrimentally on the working relationship.

The following are some key questions for the worker when developing competent practice in this area:

- In what way might my visual appearance and presentation affect the immediate engagement process with the user?
- What do I need to understand about my own values in order to practise competently?

- What are the key elements in my own personal history which might affect me in this area of work?
- What may be happening in my personal life at the moment which may affect me professionally – and in what ways?
- What do I need to do in order to ensure appropriate professional/personal boundaries?

*Making and sustaining working relationships*
These communication skills are not peculiar to the social worker/ user relationship. They are extensions in the professional context to the skills all of us need in our everyday interpersonal relationships (Egan, 1990). The process of engagement is of paramount importance to the possibility of sustaining a working relationship, and this process starts from the initial point of contact, often the written referral. Paying close attention to the written information, and considering how to initiate and achieve contact with the user, whether in person or via the telephone, is a key to effective practice. How the information is addressed, how differences are acknowledged sensitively, and in what way verbally and non-verbally the worker approaches the user are part of this process. The worker's age, gender, and other discernible characteristics will all need to be considered as part of paying attention to the immediate impact of contact (d'Ardenne and Mahtani, 1989).

Helping the users clarify their problem, tell their story, involves listening to and understanding that story in context. These elements communicate an empathic response to the user and translate that understanding into active response. An accurate perception of the user's situation and the ability to challenge assertively are part of the active response. The latter aspect is often particularly difficult for workers, who are sometimes immobilised by the complexity of different power relationships between themselves and their clients. However in the context of a sustained working relationship, challenging is often an important aspect of the work and of the process of change. Being specific and tactful, and inviting users to act on their own values, not the workers' (Egan, 1990), are fundamental characteristics of effective challenge, with clear goals in mind.

The worker may use different theoretical models to gain an overview of their working relationships, as well as the detail of them. Whatever the model, the stages of the relationship and the impact of these stages on the work need to be addressed. For example, significant losses in a user's life may complicate the sensitive ending phase of the relationship. Unfinished business, a relapse of some kind, ending too soon or not soon enough are all features of both users' and workers' difficulties at this stage. Supervision is an important resource in order for the worker to develop an overview of the work. This issue receives further attention later.

Essentially, in a brief or longer-term working relationship the worker is seeking to establish a meaningful insight with the user in the relationship between experience, feeling and behaviour. This is done through listening to and understanding both the content and process of meetings and actively using this knowledge with a view to exploring and facilitating potential change. Part of this may be to realise that change is not possible, or at least not within the time limits of a piece of work, for example in a statutory context. Again, this may be a difficult conclusion for the worker to reach and will be addressed in more detail later (Conn and Turner, 1990). The following are some key questions for the worker in developing competent practice in this area:

- Have I discussed my understanding of the users' story with them or am I making assumptions?
- Am I working at the users' pace? If not are there agency-based reasons for this which need to be explained? If not, am I moving too fast or too slowly – and for what reason?
- If I feel lost or unsure, on what do I base this? Were there things I should have done at the engagement stage?
- Am I using supervision/consultation to maintain an overview of my work? If not, for what reasons?

This is not an exhaustive list of interpersonal skills but does address key areas in developing competent practice. These core attributes have been consistently referred to in social work practice based texts, although the language used and the context around them will constantly change.

*Using authority*
The use of authority as part of good practice involves balancing several complex and delicate issues. Authority which is experienced as appropriate, contained, just, and clearly defined is not some sort of spontaneous happening. In the social worker/user relationship the power invested in the former according to role already introduces the notion of authority. Some situations (for example statutory and residential work) will involve this more strongly than others both for user and worker. Additionally there may be important visible differences between worker and user that reinforce power differentials, replicating differences in the social/political context of life outside that relationship.

Taking responsibility for appropriate use of authority needs to address these levels in order to give the users maximum opportunity to resolve their situation. Clearly establishing boundaries of the worker's role, agency function and the requirements in relation to the individual piece of work (for instance court reports and conference reports) all contribute to authority being accessibly defined.

Within these parameters, there is the personal skill of the worker in using that position in an empowering way. This implies a strong sense of self, on both a personal and a professional level, clarity about personal boundaries, as well as a genuine empathy for the user and the user's context. At the same time a professional detachment from personal and interpersonal relationships must be maintained. Using authority well draws on the skills outlined earlier in this chapter. It also requires the worker at times to contain and deal with degrees of hostility and aggression in a way which maintains professional boundaries, while assessing the degree of risk to self or other. Authority in this sense may involve containment and direct action.

Any position of authority in relation to others is open to abuses of power. This is particularly relevant in a context where workers will at times be working with vulnerable adults, young people and children. Maintaining a non-abusive position may be helped by learning from users' experiences, in written or verbal form. The following are some key questions for the worker in developing competence in this area:

- How can I tell if I am maintaining a reasonable balance (e.g. by observing user response, whether overt or covert)?
- Do I understand my role enough to use authority comfortably?
- How might any lack of confidence I feel affect my use of authority (i.e. too much or too little)?
- How might my use of authority actually or potentially replicate earlier experiences of authority figures for the user? With what possible results?
- How might my own personal experiences affect my use of professional authority?

*Working with difference*
There is a growing body of literature to refer to in this field (for example Ahmad, 1990; d'Ardenne and Mahtani, 1989; Kareem and Littlewood, 1992; Langan and Day, 1992; Oliver, 1991). Within the scope of this section we are essentially addressing both the unique experience of workers'/users' relationships, the differences between

them, and the context in which the relationships take place – the immediate, multi-disciplinary, or wider societal context.

The personal values which both client and worker bring to any encounter, based primarily on their socioeconomic, educational and cultural experiences, can influence both the process of the encounter and the content in terms of what is shared, in what way, and with what aims. The worker ostensibly has more power (though see Vass (1984) for an alternative view), delineated by the professional role, but this is not always experienced as such. For example, women in residential work often occupy an ambiguous position in the social structure. As Aymer (1992:191) suggests, 'On the one hand they must provide a private function of caring which is highly valued but on the other hand a public function which is demoralising and devalued.'

It must be the responsibility of the worker to decide how and when to address differences in the relationship. This will form part of the basis of developing an understanding from which new solutions can spring. In acknowledging the importance of making difference something that can be openly owned and talked about there is sometimes a tendency amongst those feeling less confident in this area to forget that this is a dynamic process. Once acknowledged it is somehow resolved or put to one side. Similarly to other aspects of process, difference will continue to play an important part in the life of work with a client, and needs to be consistently considered (and possibly referred to) in this way.

The impact of the wider social context, and the agency which the worker represents, will often form a key part of the individual piece of interaction. For example, in working with someone who has experienced the difficulties of migration, there are immediate issues a worker would want to consider as part of the task: loss and separation from a country, from family members, from a language commonly shared, hostility from neighbours or on the street, bureaucratic and legal difficulties, which are often mirrored in agency negotiations regarding housing, benefits, education and so on. Sensitivity to the context makes these and other questions of immediate relevance, and this widens the spectrum within which behaviour is understood. Stages of loss, dealing with hostile bureaucracies, and other hostilities, bring forth responses which can then be labelled aggressive, depressed, inadequate and so on. Viewing these as the only possible responses to an untenable situation offers a very different explanation. The following are some key questions for the worker in developing competence in this area:

- What is the context of the relationship for myself and for the user?

- How do these differ and with what potential results?
- How do my own values affect my practice when working with difference? With what potential results?
- What do I need to do within my own agency, or with other agencies, to promote competent practice in this area?

*Working in partnership: advocacy and negotiation*
These three notions may not always be seen to belong together, but they can form part of the same continuum. Both advocacy and negotiation have their place in any partnership: not consistently, but as something a person at times may be more empowered to do. In developing a professional partnership there will almost inevitably be an imbalance of power, so the notion of partnership may in itself be questionable. Notwithstanding these difficulties, being able to act as an advocate or negotiator on a user's behalf will sometimes be jointly agreed as appropriate, using position and role.

The Children Act 1989 and the National Health Service and Community Care Act 1990 have both brought the concept of working in partnership firmly on to the agenda. The paramountcy of parental responsibility as opposed to agency responsibility could be seen both as a commitment to empowering practice and as a reflection of an economic and political climate which encourages individual rather than state responsibility. This tension can have an effect on staff, who may experience a sense of cognitive dissonance: an inconsistency between their beliefs and how they should behave.

Marsh and Fisher (1992) offer five principles of working in partnership which also address issues of authority for social work intervention. The following is an adaptation of these:

(a) Investigation of problems should be with the explicit consent of the potential user, wherever possible.
(b) User agreement or a clear statutory mandate are the only basis for partnership-based intervention.
(c) The views of all relevant family members and carers are sought to inform decision-making.
(d) Services are based on negotiated agreement wherever possible rather than assumptions and/or prejudices concerning the behaviour and wishes of the users.
(e) Users should have the greatest degree of choice possible in the services offered.

The following are some key questions for the worker in developing competence in this area:

- Have I negotiated a working agreement which is clear to all parties?
- Have I included all relevant views in any decision-making process?
- How might users describe their experience of the service?
- Have I maximised the possibilities of choice in this situation?
- Am I clear about the balance between the use of authority and working in partnership in each situation? Am I maintaining that balance appropriately?

### Decision-making skills

Decision-making involves three key concepts: authority, responsibility and accountability. The appropriate use of authority was referred to earlier. This and the other two concepts should all happen as part of a process of partnership with the user. In some instances, of course, the weighting of these concepts towards the worker is considerable and has to be so in terms of agency function (e.g. child protection situations or the broader context of probation work). In others, much of the responsibility may rest with the user, as well as some of the authority to act, and a level of accountability to self, to others and/or to the agency. Working agreements should facilitate clarity in this area: who is responsible for what, in what circumstances, and to whom they are accountable.

Assessment is an example of an area of work which necessarily incorporates a decision-making function. There is a broad spectrum of assessment, from quite small pieces of work to major interventions into users' lives. The decision-making processes involved will similarly reflect the level of statutory intervention, agency and legal requirements, and any other relevant factors. Even in situations where there can be no agreement between the agency and the user about decisions made, there can at least be clarity about what they are. For example, the Department of Health guidelines on protecting children (Department of Health, 1988) offer a comprehensive guide to necessary information collation to inform the decision-making process. The results and interpretation of that information need to be available to parents/carers/children/young people wherever possible as part of the process of trying to develop working relationships. They also need to be available to other agencies, and in multi-agency situations there must be a clear understanding of different roles and clear contracts of work between departments to facilitate decision-making for workers and families (Department of Health, 1991d).

Needs-led assessments as defined by the Department of Health

(1991b; see also 1991a) address the requirements of the individual to achieve, maintain or restore an acceptable quality of life. This is, however, defined by the particular authority or care agency, so that although the concepts of choice or empowerment may ostensibly be high on the agenda, the reality of the decision-making process may be so bound by economic restraint and resource availability that shared decision-making is in reality heavily curtailed.

Coulshed (1991) emphasises the personal and professional values and assumptions which underlie any decision-making process. She places these in six categories:

1. theoretical (use of knowledge, cognitive skills, etc.);
2. economic;
3. aesthetic (personal preference);
4. social (valuing the quality of human relationships);
5. political (taking account of power balances);
6. religious (a belief in what is right or good).

These are only some of the influences on the apparently rational process of decision-making, but they indicate the complexities which are at times present to trap the unwary worker. Uncertainty, ambiguity, lack of time or reflective space, conflicting needs and values all affect the process and the outcome.

Using the skills already discussed in this chapter, weighing up sets of information, using supervision appropriately, getting advice in complex situations, all contribute to developing competent practice in what can be one of the most difficult areas of work. Some key questions for the worker to ask are as follows:

- What are the bases for any decision I might make (e.g. research findings, interviews, 'hunches')? Is this sufficient? If not, what else do I need to do?
- Have I consulted all appropriate parties, both users and other professionals?
- Is the situation about which the decision is to be made clear to all concerned?
- If clarity is problematic are the reasons for this known, and how does this inform any decision made?
- What is the element of risk involved?
- Are the decisions addressing that risk?
- How can I double-check this?

### Use and management of resources

Knowing the range of resources available to self and user is clearly a precursor to using them. This information may be readily available, or it may require a degree of effort on the part of the worker to collate an accurate picture of the resources available from public, private or voluntary sector sources in their field of work. Supervision and consultation are of paramount importance as part of a formal structure. Groups of peers, for example black workers' groups, can also be an important part of the formal structure. Informal networks of support or contacts resulting in service provision can be a creative part of the workers' vocabulary as well.

There is a further creative and empowering side to the issue of resources. Some knowledge and competence in budgeting resources in the current sociopolitical and economic context is required of social workers. The workers may themselves be able to influence the way in which resources are deployed or used, either as new possibilities, or within existing frameworks. Some key questions to ask here are as follows:

- Can I identify consistent gaps in resources for my area of work?
- If so, is there anything I could do to address this – or are there gaps in my own knowledge?
- How do I communicate the existence of possible resources to users?
- Could I do this more effectively or in a more empowering way?
- Do I use resources for myself well? How do I know this?
- Am I able to administer a budget when necessary?
- Can I argue convincingly for resources at a time of scarcity?

## Conclusion

This chapter addressed both micro and macro skills in major areas of practice. It is not an exhaustive account, but an indication of areas of skills development necessary for competent practice. Illustrative areas of competent practice can be found in more detail in the final chapter.

The divisions used here, while not arbitrary, to an extent artificially divide skills which interrelate and overlap. Cognitive skills are necessary in carrying out any of the functions of the work, for example decision-making. Making and sustaining working relationships is a cornerstone of good practice, and of carrying out agency function. These are unreachable without good interpersonal skills and an active understanding of working with difference. Sound administration underpins the whole practice structure.

Workers may at different times draw on only some of the skills mentioned, and at other times may utilise all of them. Different situations will require different skills. The spectrum of simple to extremely complex tasks will also dictate what skills are used. The context in which any of these skills is used is inherently uncertain. Uncertain because of political, legislative and organisational changes; and the uncertainty and ambiguity of the human dilemmas with which social workers become involved. The notion of skills development is not static. It is part of a dynamic process for the worker, drawing on personal experience, professional training, and learning in the work context. It will continually draw on clearly identified changes, for instance in legislation, and on the constant process of engaging with others and learning from them. Service users can be excellent trainers in skills development, if workers are willing to acknowledge this.

## References

Ahmad, B. (1990) *Black Perspectives in Social Work*. Birmingham: Venture Press.

Aymer, C. (1992) 'Women in residential work: dilemmas and ambiguities', in M. Langan and L. Day (eds), *Women, Oppression and Social Work*. London: Routledge, pp. 186–201.

Barclay, P.M. (1982) *Social Workers, their Roles and Tasks*. London: National Institute of Social Work, Bedford Square Press. (Barclay Report.)

British Association of Social Workers (1983) *Effective and Ethical Record Keeping. Report of the BASW Case Recording Project Group*. Birmingham: BASW.

CCETSW (1991) *DipSW: Rules and Requirements for the Diploma in Social Work* (Paper 30), 2nd edn. London Central Council for Education and Training in Social Work.

CCETSW (1995) *DipSW: Rules and Requirements for the Diploma in Social Work* (Paper 30), revised edn. London: Central Council for Education and Training in Social Work.

Cleaver, H. and Freeman, P. (1994) *Parental Perspectives in Cases of Suspected Child Abuse*, London: HMSO.

Conn, J. and Turner, A. (1990) 'Working with women in families', in R. Perlberg and A. Miller (eds), *Gender and Power in Families*. London: Routledge, pp. 175–95.

Coulshed, V. (1991) *Social Work Practice*, 2nd edn. London; BASW/Macmillan Education.

d'Ardenne, P. and Mahtani, A. (1989) *Transcultural Counselling in Action*. London: Sage.

Department of Health (1988) *Protecting Children: A Guide for Social Workers Undertaking a Comprehensive Assessment*. London: HMSO.

Department of Health (1989a) *Caring for People: Community Care in the Next Decade and Beyond*. London: HMSO.

Department of Health (1989b) *Working for Patients*. London: HMSO.

Department of Health (1990) *Caring for People: Policy Guidance*. London: HMSO.

Department of Health (1991a) *Care Management and Assessment*. London: HMSO.

Department of Health (1991b) *Child Abuse: A Study of Inquiry Reports 1980–1989*. London: HMSO.

Department of Health (1991c) *Patterns and Outcomes in Child Placements*. London: HMSO.

Department of Health (1991d) *Working Together under the Children Act 1989*. London: HMSO.

Doel, M. and Lawson, B. (1986) 'Open records: the client's right to partnership', *British Journal of Social Work*, 16: 407–30.

Egan, G. (1990) *The Skilled Helper* 4th edn. Pacific Grove: Brooks/Cole.

Ford, K. and Jones, A. (1987) *Student Supervision*. London: BASW/Macmillan.

Gibbons, J. (ed.) (1993) *The Children Act 1989 and Family Support: Principles into Practice*. London: HMSO.

Home Office, Department of Health and Welsh Office (1995) *National Standards for the Supervision of Offenders in the Community*. London: Home Office Probation Division.

Kareem, J. and Littlewood, R. (1992) *Intercultural Therapy*. Oxford: Blackwell Scientific Publications.

Langan, M. and Day, L. (1992) *Women, Oppression and Social Work*. London: Routledge.

Little, M. and Gibbons, J. (1993) 'Predicting the rate of children on the child protection register', *Research, Policy and Planning*, 10: 15–18.

McIvor, G. (1992) *Sentence to Serve*. Aldershot: Avebury.

Marsh, P. and Fisher, M. (1992) *Good Intentions: Developing Partnership in Social Services*. York: Joseph Rowntree Foundation.

Oliver, J. (ed.) (1991) *Disabled People and Disabling Environments*. London: Jessica Kingsley.

Orme, J. and Glastonbury, B. (1993) *Care Management*. London: BASW/Macmillan.

Ovretveit, J. (1986) *Improving Social Work Records and Practice*. Birmingham: BASW.

Perlberg, R. and Miller, A. (eds) (1990) *Gender and Power in Families*. London: Routledge.

Raynor, P. (1988) *Probation as an Alternative to Custody: A Case Study*. Aldershot: Gower.

Seebohm, I. (1968) *Report of the Committee on Local Authority and Allied Services*. London: HMSO.

Vass, A.A. (1984) *Sentence to Labour: Close Encounters with a Prison Substitute*. St Ives: Venus Academica.

Vass, A.A. (1990) *Alternatives to Prison: Punishment, Custody and the Community*. London: Sage.

# 4

# Social Work with Children and Families

More than any other specialism within the profession, social work with children and families has received detailed media attention and been subjected to much public debate and scrutiny. Many social workers will be aware that, particularly within child protection work, the opinions expressed about practitioners have been unfavourable (Franklin and Parton, 1991).

In essence, two types of opinions are expressed. First that social workers do too little, too late. When a child dies at the hands of its carers, public inquiries are instigated to explore the role of welfare services, especially social work, in failing to protect the child (Department of Health, 1982, 1991a). Whether or not the inquiries reach conclusions about professional negligence or individual culpability, the publicity given by the media often focuses on one social worker, who is presented as naive, gullible, blameworthy and in some circumstances committing murder by proxy (Ruddock, 1991). The other opinion, a polar opposite of the first, is that social workers do too much, too soon. This is most sharply expressed via other public inquiries, for example in Cleveland (DHSS, 1988) where child sexual abuse was the issue, or in the Orkney Isles where ritualised abuse was suspected. In these cases dawn raids to remove children from their homes, denial of contact between children and their carers and the provision of inexpert evidence for legal proceedings have been highlighted and criticised.

Whereas in the first example social workers are presented as weak and ineffectual, in the second they are seen as draconian, paying little regard to the sanctity of family life. In the eyes of the media at present those social workers working with children and families are 'damned if they do and damned if they don't' (Preston-Shoot and Agass, 1990).

Lack of care and an uncritical wish for control create a composite picture of professional incompetence. Within the profession itself, stress is experienced as high and the rewards few (Audit Commission, 1994: para. 179), to some extent continuing the 'confusion compounded by uncertainty' noted over a decade ago by the Barclay Committee when reviewing the roles and tasks of social workers (Barclay, 1982).

A second contextual factor which adds to the confusion and uncertainty stems from the fact that social work with children and families is mainly located within, or funded by, local government. Here, diminished resources and increased demand collide, and only a skeletal version of the original post-World War II idea of welfare services remains. Perhaps the most alarming impact on the relationships between social workers and service users in this climate is that the profession's capacity to care recedes while there is a simultaneous growth in its statutory, more controlling functions. This is illustrated in the following example.

**Case example**

Cathy Simms, a lone parent with three children, refers herself to the social services department. She says to the duty social worker that she is finding it difficult to control her 10-year-old daughter, Susan. She describes truanting from school, Susan hitting her younger brother and sister and having nightmares which are frequent. Susan is occasionally enuretic. She says she wants to go and live with her father, who left the family nine months ago. Susan's father gives no financial support to Cathy. She says she has no money for food and her Income Support has been spent. Fuel debts have mounted and disconnection is threatened. She wants financial help, day care for the younger children so that she can return to work, and someone to 'look' at her daughter's behaviour.

The social worker completes an application for day care, only to be told by the childminding adviser that there is a long waiting list for day-care places. Cathy agrees to a referral to the local Child Guidance Unit (CGU) for the family to be seen in relation to Susan's behaviour. The CGU accepts the referral on the under-standing that an appointment may be delayed by several weeks due to staff shortages. The fuel board insists that a substantial amount of the debt is cleared immediately before the threat of disconnection is withdrawn. The Department of Social Security agrees to make a lump-sum payment to the fuel board if Cathy agrees that some money is deducted each week from her benefits until the debt is cleared. Reluctantly Cathy accepts this, knowing that it will place a greater pressure on the family's capacity to cope. The social worker makes out a small grant to Cathy for food (Children Act 1989: section 17) and promises to let her know about the day care as soon as a place becomes available.

A week later a teacher from Susan's school contacts social services to say that Susan has returned to school after an absence of several days. A small circular mark, like a cigarette burn, has been noted on her arm. She is frightened to go home and says that her mother is angry. A social worker visits the home and finds Cathy agitated and verbally abusive, admitting to having hurt Susan but saying that she can no longer tolerate her daughter's behaviour. She says that she will hurt Susan again if she needs to, and is angry at the unwarranted intrusion into her life only a few days after not receiving the help that she needed. The social worker concludes that Susan is at risk of further harm at the hands of her mother and should not return home. In consultation with the senior social worker an application is made to a local magistrates' court for an Emergency Protection Order (Children Act 1989: section 44).

Susan is placed with foster carers. The social services department considers whether any further legal steps need to be taken to protect the children in the family. A child protection case conference is convened to evaluate risk to the children. Cathy is invited but does not attend. Instead she takes her grievances against the department to a local newspaper, which publishes another item on bureaucratic abuse of natural justice, citing Cathy's case as an example.

In this bleak but not unfamiliar scenario a connecting pattern of abuse emerges. Not only does the mother abuse the daughter, taking control beyond reasonable limits, but the 'welfare' is seen to abuse her rights as a parent in a similar manner and is in turn caricatured and criticised by the media. It is this ebb and flow of hostile and competitive exchanges between parents and social workers that is presented to the outside world as standard social work practice. In this narrow scope of analysis individuals are apportioned blame – 'a bad parent', 'the SS worker' – while the context in which the actions and reactions have taken place is seldom paid the attention it deserves. Nor for that matter is much attention given to the good practice that continues to exist despite resource constraints and bad press.

This chapter, in concerning itself with issues of competence, focuses by and large not on an idealised standard of practice but on the ways in which practitioners can achieve clarity of purpose and consistency in offering a high-quality service to users. This is done via identifying the importance in childcare work of being child-centred and working in partnership with carers. These principles, spelt out directly by recent Department of Health guidance and regulations (e.g. Department of Health, 1990) and enshrined in the Children Act 1989, are not new to social work, and have indeed been informed by practice wisdom accumulated by practitioners and policy-makers within the profession over the last half-century (see Jordan, 1984). To some extent they underline a value position in the profession of user involvement (Marsh and Fisher, 1992) and client empowerment (Ward and Mullender, 1991) as an active counter-point to the abuses of professional power noted by the tabloid press and some recent inspections of services for children and families (Social Services Inspectorate, 1993). Here we accept the thesis that competence lies in viewing the child as 'a person and not an object of concern' (DHSS, 1988: 245), reflecting to a significant degree the welfare principles set out in section 1 of the Children Act 1989. In fact so much of social work with children and families is now linked to the Children Act 1989 that it is best, in describing the duties, roles and responsibilities of workers, to be explicit about their connections with the legislation. In principle at least, the focus of work is on three broad areas: first, in offering a preventative service to families caring for vulnerable children; secondly, the investigation of harm to children, and the use of child protection procedures; thirdly, the use of statutory measures to remove children from home and provide substitute care with foster parents or in residential units.

Overall the intention of the legislators has been to pick up and act upon a number of important issues within each of these areas in order to reinforce organisational and individual professional competence. So, for example, prevention of family breakdown by alleviating social and material deprivation is amplified and specified. In child protection, emphasis is placed on working cooperatively with adult carers where possible rather than competing with them to care for a child. Thirdly, in relation to children being looked after by the local authority, continuity of contact with their community of origin is highlighted. These issues are discussed below. Connections between the ways in which parents, social workers and others can work together in caring for vulnerable children are made. Points at which consensus begins to diminish and conflict arises are high-lighted.

**Preventative services**

The Children Act 1989 introduced a new legislative framework for family support, based on a duty to provide services for children in need and their families, in order to prevent family breakdown (Part III and schedule 2). A child is seen as being in need if, broadly speaking,

> s/he is unlikely to achieve or maintain a reasonable standard of health (physical and mental) or development (physical, intel-lectual, emotional, social or behavioural), unless the local authority provides help in some way; *or* if s/he is disabled (see section 17 (10)).

A substantial body of research now exists linking poverty to the risk of children being received into the system of public care (see Audit Commission, 1994).

For example, Gibbons (1991) confirms that families experiencing childcare problems which had been referred to social services were distinguishable from the general run of families along a number of dimensions, most notably social disadvantage and deprivation, personal vulnerability, and lack of social support. Bebbington and Miles (1988) examined the circumstances and backgrounds of children coming into care and found that the following accumulation of factors increases the chances of being 'looked after' at some time before the age of 17.

| CHILD 'A' | CHILD 'B' |
|---|---|
| Aged 5 to 9 | Aged 5 to 9 |
| No dependence on state benefits | Household head gets Income Support |
| Two-parent family | Single-adult household |
| Three or fewer children | Four or more children |
| White | Mixed racial origin |
| Owner-occupier home | Privately rented home |
| More rooms than people | One or more persons per room |

*Odds of being 'looked after'*

| 1 in 7,000 | 1 in 10 |
|---|---|

(*Source*: Bebbington and Miles, 1988)

Holman (1988) is clear that in such circumstances social workers can and should take a proactive role in alleviating poverty by offering, as a first step in attempting to give a competent service, a number of interventions or services, which all local authorities have the power to provide. Some of these are listed below (although see Brayne and Martin, 1990 for a fuller list).

- Financial help (Children Act 1989, section 17 (6)) or 'assistance in kind'. Generally this means that families can turn to social services departments if they run out of money or food or clothing for their children when the children going without these things would endure unreasonable hardship. Payments of small grants or loans can be made, but no family in receipt of Income Support or Family Credit is liable for any repayment (Children Act 1989, section 17 (9)).
- The provision of advice, guidance and counselling. In their day-to-day work social workers may be asked to advise, guide and

counsel people with a variety of problems. In defining specific areas of work under these broad headings, social workers may directly intervene, refer on to specialist help, or work alongside specialist workers in other professions in achieving jointly identified goals.

Local authorities, via their social services departments (SSDs), are encouraged to provide 'occupational, social, cultural and recreational activities' for children and their families. The guidance and regulations to the Children Act 1989, volume 2, focus on family support and day care for young children (Department of Health, 1991d: vol. 2). Here it is suggested that if local authorities do not already do so, a range of services should be provided in order to prevent children coming into care. For example:

- day care offered by childminders or nurseries (which the SSD must inspect, register and support on a regular basis);
- befriending schemes or parent and toddler groups for isolated parents;
- toy libraries;
- drop-in centres where members of a locality can meet;
- family centres where therapeutic work can take place in improving parenting skills;
- home helps or family aides who can offer parents practical help in running the household, especially if a parent is ill or if a child has disabilities which place an excessive burden of care on a parent;
- accommodation (section 22 (2)). In many ways this is a new and innovative provision. The Act recognises that sometimes, perhaps for short periods, parents and children need to live apart from each other, particularly when the situation at home reaches a crisis point and living together may result in harm to or lack of care for the child. Parents are encouraged to apply to local authority SSDs for respite from their task of parenting. They can withdraw their children from substitute care at any time they choose under this arrangement (in previous legislation this was not always the case, and children drifted along on a 'voluntary' basis until further statutory action was taken by SSDs to exert control over their lives).

Despite the legislators giving the above definition and outlining services to meet need, Tunstill (1992) is clear that the Act stops some way short of compelling local authorities to work preventatively. Considerable discretion is built into the ways in which the legislation itself and the guidance and regulations stemming from it are interpreted. For example, volume 2 of the *Guidance and Regulations* on family support and day care states that:

> This guidance does not lay down firm criteria or set general priorities because the Act requires each authority to decide their own level and scale of services appropriate to the children in need in their area. (Department of Health, 1991d: para. 2.4)

And further on:

> Local authorities are not expected to meet every individual need, but they are expected to identify the extent of need and then to make decisions on the priorities for service provision in the context of that information and their statutory duties (Department of Health, 1991d: para. 2.11).

Given this flexibility, lack of organisational competence has been discovered by the Audit Commission (1994) which notes, amongst its various concerns, that little systematic identification of the extent of relative need has taken place in Britain in the 1990s, by either health or social services. This has resulted in resources not being targeted effectively, and in more generally available provisions not being used effectively. Objectives of services are frequently vague and outcomes unclear, often leading to reactive rather than pro-active planning and practice; working in partnership with service users, whilst acknowledged in principle, is not fully implemented in practice. Giller (1993) acknowledges that agencies and workers appear to be working at what he terms a tertiary rather than primary level of prevention, illustrating these levels as shown in Table 4.1.

In commenting further on this division in the levels of prevention Rose (1993) notes the existence of a number of interrelated obstacles which impede the effective development of family support services. For example, prevention is not prioritised in relation to protection. Responding to referrals of child abuse has become a key organising factor of the culture of professional practice, mediated to some extent by unfavourable media coverage. Where this type of work is recognised as having its own validity, existing within clearer and specific guidelines, preventative work is seen as somehow old-fashioned, not 'real work' which attracts status and power, and as having vague aims and processes. Difficulties in evaluating its cost-effectiveness are highlighted. In a climate of financial uncertainty, where short-term objectives take precedence over developing longer-term policies, services and strategies, it is seen as slow to build up. Lack of workload management schemes which actively encourage workers to balance preventative work with child protection work are missing or sketchily addressed.

Given these types of obstacles the messages from research, which

Table 4.1 *Levels of prevention*

| Key features | Primary | Secondary | Tertiary |
|---|---|---|---|
| Practice ideology | • developmental<br>• change system rather than people<br>• empowerment | • welfare<br>• help for the client<br>• assessment of need | • judicial<br>• rescue the victim<br>• punish the villain |
| Stage of problem development (assessment of risk and/or need) | • Low or containable risk<br>• problems common to many (vulnerable groups)<br>• citizens rather than clients | • low/medium risk but high perceived need<br>• acute crisis or early stage of problem<br>• short-term client | • chronic problems<br>• high risk of harm to self or other<br>• high need for protection of child<br>• perception of parental need may be low |
| Major unit of need | • localities<br>• vulnerable groups | • nuclear family | • individual family members perceived as problematic or in need of rescue or protection |
| Principal targets of intervention | • welfare institutions<br>• community networks<br>• social policy | • family systems<br>• support networks<br>• welfare institution | • personal change |

| | | |
|---|---|---|
| Objectives of intervention | • reallocation of resources<br>• redistribution of power/control over resources (inc. resources of social work agencies)<br>• increased rights for disadvantaged groups | • enhanced family functioning<br>• enhanced support network<br>• family's increased awareness and motivation to make use of existing resources<br>• welfare institutions more responsive to people's needs | • better-adjusted, less deviant individuals; self-supporting families |
| Dominant mode of practice | • community action<br>• community development<br>• community social work | • generic multi-role practitioner<br>• social care planning<br>• social casework | • individual casework<br>• treatment or therapy |

*Source:* Giller, 1993

highlights organisational and practice competence with regard to preventative work, suggest that the provisions as outlined in the Children Act 1989 (see above) do significantly contribute to children being cared for by their families of origin (see, for example, Benzeval and Judge, 1992; Cox et al., 1992; Hardiker, 1992; Holman, 1989; Gibbons, 1992). However, there is no simple correlation between availability of resources and the ways that professionals act in using them to enable families to continue caring for their children. Rather there is evidence to suggest that, within limits, practitioners can carry out effective preventative work within organisations where resources are limited, as long as they can map out the following and are as clear as possible about how to achieve them, within the context in which they work:

● *what* it is they and others are seeking to prevent from happening;
● *how* the agreed resolutions are going to be put into effect;
● *who* takes appropriate responsibility, together with or separately from others, in securing available resources or finances;
● *why* the map created by identifying the above is in line with the best interests of the child within the overall framework of prevention;
● *when* the aim(s) of intervention are achieved, as evidenced by changes in people's behaviour and/or circumstances against criteria which have been specified or modified in agreement between the parties concerned.

Prevention is not created unilaterally by a single worker. The action by a worker in identifying and seeking prevention is part of a collective effort by a number of people located within the informal and formal networks of care surrounding vulnerable children. Here a greater degree of consensus between these people – on the definition of need, targets of intervention and how those targets are to be achieved within a strategically coherent framework – still needs to be reached.

### Child protection

Issues of working together are very much to the fore in investigating and dealing with children who have been abused or neglected. In part this is because these children form a natural sub-group of the broader population of children in need. Also, and significantly, public scrutiny of the lives of children who have been caught in the net of child protection has led to the conclusion that at times cooperation between carers and workers has been low whilst criticism, conflict and competition have been high (Department of

Health, 1991a). Some of the tensions inherent in carers, social workers and other professions working together are examined below.

One aspect of this tension is the definition of abuse itself. Determining what is and is not abusive behaviour is seldom possible without reference to the context in which the behaviour takes place (Department of Health, 1995). Equally, societal perspectives of what constitutes abusive behaviour may change over time and across racial and cultural boundaries (Parton, 1985; Ahmad, 1990). Sometimes, perhaps on most occasions that child protection investigations take place, it may only be possible to think about people having a perspective on child abuse as opposed to a conclusive or unassailable definition. Given the capacity for definitions to be influenced in this way, competence in the workers may rest in part on their ability to maintain a focus of concern about the severity and chronicity of behaviours, bearing in mind that a few behaviours universally and over time remain abusive. For example, it may be easier to develop consensus on the notion that a carer stubbing out a cigarette on a child repeatedly is abusive in comparison to smacking them or being naked in their company. Shouting at a child may not in itself constitute abuse, but over time, in a context which is low in warmth and high on criticism of the child, it may lead to emotional harm. Competent practice thus involves having a clear understanding of both the point at which behaviour by a parent becomes maltreatment and the point at which such behaviour requires professional intervention. In other words, the competent professional is able to describe a threshold for intervention. Latterly in Britain such thresholds have been set in a number of ways, for example by laying down child protection procedures, creating categories of abuse under which children can be registered and identifying the type and quality of working relationships which may lead to better protection of children.

There has been a substantial growth in the last few years in the number of children who have been the focus of child protection investigation and registration. For example in 1986 there were 15,000 children's names on child protection registers in England and Wales (Taylor, 1989). The latest survey in England alone indicates that the total had reached 38,600 by the end of 1992 (Department of Health, 1993), a prevalence rate of 3.5 children per thousand aged 18 years or under. Of these, approximately 28,000 were children of school age and 16,000 of them had been registered in the year preceding the survey. There is currently a substantial amount of research commissioned by the Department of Health which provides an insight into children, child abuse and child protection. A recent fairly conservative estimate suggests that out of the 11 million children living in England and Wales, about 650,000 live in an environment which poses a risk to their health and development (Smith and Bentovim, 1994). About 190 of them die each year, and the cause of death can reasonably be attributed to neglect or abuse by the carer (Department of Health, 1993). About 200,000 are referred to child protection systems. Seventy-five per cent of these referrals are investigated further. Whilst a minority (1,400) are compulsorily removed, about 50,000 are the subject of a case conference; 25,000 of these have their names placed on the child protection register.

Importantly, when children are registered, a variety of factors beyond the information relating to the child and family influence the registration process. For example, if the ratio of social workers to residents is low in a given locality, or if day care, family support services or play group provisions are poor, where unemployment is high as is the number of children within the public care system, and when organisations have no specialist child protection posts and no specific criteria for removing names from the register, then the rates of registration are higher than in localities where these conditions apply less strongly (Little and Gibbons, 1993).

Equally important, Gibbons et al. (1993) have identified the following general characteristics among children and families investigated. From a sample of nearly 2,000 cases in 1992 in England and Wales over one-third (36 per cent) were headed by a lone parent, 57 per cent lacked a wage earner, 54 per cent of heads of households were dependent on Income Support, in 27 per cent of families domestic violence was experienced, and in 13 per cent mental illness of parent was a feature. They also found that 15 per cent of abusing parents had a known history of being abused as children themselves, that 65 per cent of children investigated were already known to social services, in 45 per cent of children investigated a previous investigation had taken place, in 99 per cent of cases the perpetrator was already known to the child and that 90 per cent of adults under investigation were involved in daily care of the child. Black and Asian families were over-represented among referrals for physical injury and under-represented for sexual abuse.

Drawing conclusions from such features and conditions in terms of predicting child abuse remains difficult, partly because research has yet to establish more than a lukewarm connection between the existence of such conditions and the inevitability of harm to a child. It is one thing to assert that the characteristics and circumstances of children dealt with under child protection procedures differ from those of families and children living in England and Wales as a whole; it is quite another to say that they are typical of all families within which children are maltreated (Mitchell, 1989). As Parton (1986: 525) has pointed out, 'Whatever is done prediction rates rise no higher than two wrong judgements for every right judgement. The empirical support for the prediction of violence is very poor.'

What does become clear however is that, by and large, social workers are likely to focus their investigations on those who are most vulnerable and materially disadvantaged. The implications for competent practice may lie in recognising and assessing the degree to which contextual factors contribute to the abusive behaviour and the degree to which change in such circumstances is necessary and possible, while identifying social workers' own and others' responsibilities as specifically as possible in relation to such change.

**Parental involvement in child protection**

Parents can feel overwhelmed by the process of investigation and express alienation, anger and disempowerment about the decisions being taken (Brazil and Steward, 1992; Thoburn et al., 1993). There is a shift in the relationship between parents and social workers from one in which the possibility of care and cooperation are excluded and the probabilities of control and competition between them highlighted. At least that is how it must seem to the parents involved in the process (Prosser, 1992). From a social work point of view, investigations are reported as being stressful and anxiety-provoking affairs (Glaser and Frosh, 1988; Dale et al., 1986) where competent practice is in jeopardy. The social workers' task is not simply to cope with their own and other people's strong feelings but also, as Furniss (1991) notes, to be able to:

• clarify and be specific about the reasons for concerns leading to the investigation. They should be able to acknowledge the strength of feeling about the process of investigation with parents and children;
• explain their statutory responsibilities in a comprehensible way either verbally or in writing or by using official interpreters where necessary;
• explain the roles and duties of workers from other agencies, where necessary;
• explore the parents' own legal rights either with regard to making representations or complaints during the process or, for example, in gaining access to official records made during the course of the investigations;

- be open, honest and authoritative, particularly in stressing that the welfare of the child is the overriding factor guiding child protection work;
- inform parents about what is going to happen, how long it will take, step by step. This process of review and planning may need to happen continuously;
- inform parents about their attendance at case conferences and discuss what help could be offered to them in putting their views across. If parents will not attend, then arrangements need to be made to have their views expressed;
- help parents articulate their own abilities and strengths and solutions with regard to protection and care for their child. Especially in cases of sexual abuse the non-abusing carer (often the mother) is a vital contributor to the future safety and welfare of the child.

Guidelines developed by a number of social services departments remind their investigative staff that they should undertake child protection work in partnership with parents where possible, reflecting the *Working Together* guidelines' comment that

> it cannot be emphasised too strongly that involvement of children and adults in [child protection work] will not be effective unless they are fully involved from the outset in all stages of the process, and unless from the time of referral there is as much openness and honesty as possible between families and professionals. (Department of Health 1991c: 43, para. 6.11)

Thoburn et al. (1993) are clear that partnership with parents of children is *most* likely to work if the following conditions prevail.

- There is a single episode of abuse.
- Neglect is an issue but not seen as premeditated.
- Sexual abuse has occurred but the perpetrator is no longer living in the home.
- The abuse is related to a parent's episodic mental illness or related to a recognised stress factor.
- The parent is not implicated in the alleged abuse or neglect.
- The parent is not under suspicion of having failed to protect the child.
- The parent accepts that there is a problem.
- The parent and the social worker agree about the nature and degree of the abuse/neglect.
- The parent welcomes social work help.

Conversely, partnership is *hardest* to establish when:

- the abuse is persistent, severe or organised and where the alleged abuser still lives at home;
- the parent has a record of violence or threatening behaviour;
- the parent denies that abuse has taken place;
- the parent takes no responsibility for abuse or neglect;
- the parent rejects social work help;
- the parent cannot agree with the social worker on what has happened or what to do about it.

These researchers go to some lengths to confirm that, rather like the definition of abuse itself, partnership is not an absolute concept which is either present or absent in effective working relationships. Instead it is one end of a continuum, which ranges from non-involvement in the decision-making processes to carers being treated as equal parties from the beginning to the end of the intervention. The map they delineate above offers a competent worker the opportunity to clarify some of the significant prevailing conditions which allow carers and others to have a voice within the system, but does not constitute a predictive tool in the sense of offering absolute certainty. Competence becomes associated with using the above findings meaningfully in a context which is inherently uncertain and complex, where perhaps the need to be certain is high and confidence and morale low. In our view a good measure of competence is the worker's capacity to remain confident in dealing with uncertainty, using available knowledge within the limits of its relevance to the specific context in which s/he is working.

This can also be said about Farmer and Owen's (1993) research, which indicates that from the start of the investigative process the potential for alienating carers and children is minimised by workers who can name and contain feelings of competition, blame, fear, anger and lack of trust. Commonly, carers and children express relief at being treated kindly, where respect is maintained and the importance of being cared for as people is emphasised. Workers are appreciated when they do more than simply reiterate their statutory responsibilities; where they provide clear information about processes and aims, make investigations feel less like interrogations, involve people as fully as possible, and identify and provide resources appropriate to a comprehensive assessment of the abusing behaviour in context.

In a sense these findings act as guidelines in clarifying the notion that it is not just a matter of what a competent social worker does; importantly, it is how s/he acts that makes a difference in terms of clients' views. This connection between the what and the how of competence is also apparent in the arena of substitute care.

**Substitute care**

In the majority of cases children remain at home while services are provided, but instances do arise where they may need to be temporarily or permanently removed for their own safety and protection from circumstances in which they are likely to suffer significant harm. A child can be removed compulsorily from home using the new legislation in a specific number of ways – by obtaining an Emergency Protection Order (EPO), an Interim Care Order (ICO) or a full Care Order (CO) – although the guidance and regulations are at pains to point out that going to court should be a last resort, when all possible avenues of cooperative work between carers and workers are exhausted.

The Children Act 1989 is silent on what constitutes significance within the phrase 'significant harm' and no one is yet certain how the courts will interpret its meaning. What is clear is that harm is defined, as Allen (1990:109) explains, in these terms:

> Ill-treatment or impairment of health and development [section 31 (9)]. The interpretation of significant turns on the child's health or development being compared with that which could reasonably be expected of a similar child (i.e. of the same age, characteristics etc.).

If an application for an order is made by the social services department or other parties the court is duty bound within the framework of the Act to ask itself whether making an order is the only way to deal with the child's best interests, or indeed whether judicial intervention is necessary at all. The Children Act 1989 puts it thus (section 1 (1)):

> When a court determines any question with respect to the upbringing of a child, the child's welfare shall be the court's paramount consideration.

The idea here is that the court should remain child centred, acting, as it were, as the ultimate good parent in settling issues others may have competed over and failed to agree on. As such it would be reasonable to expect the court to scrutinise very carefully how child centred the parties represented in the case are or are prepared to be. The court would consider the following factors when making its decision about granting an order of whatever type; this is referred to as the *welfare checklist*:

A  The ascertainable wishes and feelings of the child concerned (considered in the light of his/her age and understanding).
B  His/her physical, emotional and educational needs.
C  The likely effect on him/her of any changes in circumstances.
D  His/her age, sex, background and any characteristic of his[/hers] which the court considers relevant.

E   Any harm which s/he has suffered or is at risk of suffering.
F   How capable each of his/her parents, and any other persons in relation to whom the court considers the question to be relevant, is on meeting his/her needs.
G   The range of powers available to the court under the 1989 Act in the proceedings in question. (section 1 (3))

Allen (1990) comments that the checklist is not particularly novel in that it is modelled on principles existing in previous legislation and current ideas about competent social work practice. In demonstrating competence in court, social workers will need to show to the court's satisfaction that the above factors have been attended to in their preparation for applications which are being considered. They will ordinarily be expected to show what they have attempted to do in terms of the presenting issues on a voluntary basis with carers, how they have attempted to work in partnership, why this has not been possible, and the likely effect on the child of a court order not being made. They should also have discussed the implications of their actions fully with all relevant parties.

Research into the experiences of children entering the care system, summarised in *Patterns and Outcomes in Child Placement* (Department of Health, 1991b) has highlighted the significance of their maintaining contact with their natural families and communities of origin (Millham et al., 1986: Packman et al., 1986) while in substitute care. Other research has reinforced the message that children in need of care are not necessarily characteristically children whose parents were abusive or neglectful (Rowe et al., 1989). Rather it has confirmed a strong link between admissions and material crises (precipitated by homelessness, unemployment, financial debt) or behavioural problems, with parents motivated by their children's welfare and social workers responding in a supportive manner by negotiation and agreement.

Continuity of contact at a time of necessary change has been addressed by the new legislation. For example the 1989 Act encourages the placement of a child with a person connected with that child: a family member or relative or other suitable persons (section 23 (6)); it states that the accommodation offered should be, so far as is reasonably practicable and consistent with the child's welfare, near the child's home and that siblings should be accommodated together (section 23 (7)). If a child has disabilities, arrangements need to be made to offer suitable accommodation. Similarly, due consideration needs to be given to how best a child's needs are to be met in relation to religion, race, culture and language (section 22) when finding a suitable placement.

There is explicit recognition that competent social work practice involves continued consideration, via regular reviews of children in care, of the possibility of returning home. So once a child is in care no matter for what length of time (for up to eight days with an Emergency Protection Order, or up to 18 years of age with a Care Order) contact with parents or those with parental responsibilities should whenever possible continue unless clear evidence emerges that this is detrimental to the child's well-being. The hasty removal of children by social workers to the care of people whom they do not know, living in an area which is unfamiliar to them, ought to become a thing of the past used knowingly and justifiably only when circumstances dictate that this course of action is necessary.

There is also a recognition of something that social workers and many parents have been aware of for some time – that the trauma of enforced separation, no matter how dire the circumstances from which a child is removed, can worry and preoccupy children in a way which undermines their ability and educational potential. Similarly, moving children frequently from one placement to another leads to their becoming disruptive and hard to care for. The regulations require local authorities to carry out a number of tasks. These are:

1   Notify the local education authority if a child is based in its area.
2   Recognise that a school needs to have as much information as possible about the child prior to his or her starting with them.
3   If a child is looked after by substitute carers then it is the social worker's responsibility to initiate contact between them and the school if it does not already exist.
4   The social worker should monitor the child's educational progress and general welfare by maintaining direct contact with the school, the carers, and via school reports sent to the carers. The social worker should be clear about access to specialist services within the local authority's educational provisions in order to enlist their help whenever necessary on behalf of the child.
5   The natural parents may themselves wish to contact the school or continue to play some part in the child's education. The social worker should work with the school and parent in establishing what this means in practice.
6   The social worker should help the parents exercise their rights under the statementing process.

Residential workers in children's homes are reminded of their responsibilities in providing support and encouragement beyond that which may be given by a caring parent (Department of Health, 1991e:23) to the people in their care. What the guidance and regulations do not comment on – and arguably this is beyond their remit – is that the conflicts and contradictions that have already been discussed in relation to parents, teachers and social workers and those inherent within the legislative framework can and do draw in foster carers and residential workers. Robinson (1978) and the Barclay Report (1982) both note that social workers should actively support substitute carers in their difficult task of helping children in need. Yet in many respects support may not be a straightforward process. Substitute carers, in building attachments to children, may compete with social workers in owning or disowning them. Like social workers they may pay more attention to the care-giving and domestic tasks on behalf of a child than to the child's educational attainments (Prosser, 1978). It may be difficult for them to move away from being home-centred people or, as Jackson (1989:141) argues, to 'offer much intellectual stimulation . . . or deal effectively with schools and teachers'. Berridge (1985:96) paints a graphic picture of the child coming home from school bursting to recount the day's events, 'only to find adult attention firmly focused on the chip pan and the frozen fish fingers'.

Bald (1982) describes how hard it is to persuade care staff to devote ten minutes a day to helping children with their reading. Millham et al. (1986) note how few substitute carers have themselves had satisfactory or successful experiences of education. Jackson (1989:142) summarises the context thus:

> In these circumstances it is hardly surprising that staff may have difficulty in relating to school teachers or in asserting their own judgement of a child's ability and needs in the face of a presumed expert. In addition they may be inclined to play down the importance of school attendance and gloss over difficulties, not expecting that the children in their charge will do any better than themselves.

Given these circumstances, specialist help may need to be made available to children in care in order to improve their educational abilities. Jackson (1989) describes a successful effort in inter-professional cooperation – the recruitment by a residential home of an educational liaison officer, a former teacher with intimate knowledge of local schools. Jackson (1989:148) goes on to add:

> her main task was to act as an intermediary and interpreter between care staff, children and teachers. In this her activities were similar to those which any concerned parent would take in support of their own children, with the difference that for children in residential care from disturbed backgrounds the monitoring and intervention required are almost continuous. . . . One measure of her success was the fact that no child had been suspended from school since her appointment, something which had previously been an almost weekly occurrence. . . . As a teacher

herself she was equally concerned with matters of academic achievement. . . . This transformed the children's feelings about going to school, knowing that they could hand in acceptable pieces of work.

This type of innovative work is unusual, because extra funds need to be made available in order to sustain it. A more familiar scenario at present is that foster carers and residential workers continue to feel undervalued and underpaid. For example the National Foster Care Association has drawn attention to the fact that foster parents looking after a young child are usually paid less than the weekly cost of kennelling a dog (NFCA, 1992). In substitute care, as much as in preventative work and in the protection of children from harm, issues of quality and quantity and care and control go hand in hand.

One conclusion that emerges is that the quality of care provided for children in need depends, to perhaps a substantial extent, not simply on workers and others following guidance and regulations as laid down by the Department of Health, but also on an increase in the provision of financial and material resources. In other words, professional competence in substitute care, as in other areas of social work with children and families, connects with and is mitigated by the context in which it is located.

**Looking to the future**

Considering what lies ahead in social work with children and families, there is a growing sense of the profession going back to the future. On the one hand the Children Act 1989 is clearly modelled on egalitarian principles, confirming notions of working in partnership with carers and emphasising the need to maintain children with their families. On the other hand increasing demand in relation to available resources since the late 1970s has resulted in the safety net of welfare provisions looking threadbare. The ends defined within the Children Act, which, as we have noted, reinforce the notion of professionally competent behaviour, may not be easy to achieve given the means available to social workers. Given this mismatch between principles and reality, some uncertainties arise for and within the profession in the future.

Two questions remain difficult to answer. First, how well will social workers provide the services necessary, as defined in the Children Act, to promote the notion of families caring for their own children? Secondly, how well will social workers feel cared for by those who define what they should do?

There is after all a parallel between the ways in which social workers work with families, and the ways in which they feel supported by the state in the formulation of social policy and legislation. We could pursue Gibbons's (1992:3) definition of good parenting – 'predictable, available, sensitive and responsive care-taking within a structured and responsive home environment' – and seek to apply it to the profession's relationship with the state. Here, it may be argued, the state's lack of consistency and clarity in the provision of welfare has resulted, in part at least, in a failure in its role as *parens patriae*. This in turn has led to confusion and uncertainty within social work about how best to be a good enough carer to those in need, and jeopardised the notion of competence. The recipients of services would confirm that they have at times felt the profession to be abusive of its responsibilities (Prosser, 1992).

Whilst all three parties – parents, professionals and policy-makers – may continue to argue that they have the best interests of children at heart, their arguing may disguise the complex nature of their responsibilities towards children in need and the gaps that exist between what they say ought to be done and how they end up doing it. Dissonance may continue to exist. For social workers, part of the challenge of maintaining competent practice may lie in recognising the source and impact of such dissonance on their capacities to remain balanced, available, sensitive and responsive in helping children and families in need.

## References

Ahmad, B. (1990) *Black Perspectives in Social Work*. Birmingham: Venture Press.

Allen, N. (1990) *Making Sense of the Children Act 1989*. Harlow: Longman.

Audit Commission (1994) *Seen But Not Heard. Co-ordinating Community Child Health and Social Services for Children in Need*. London: HMSO.

Bald, H. (1982) 'Children in care need books', *Concern*, 44: 18–21.

Barclay, P.M. (1982) *Social Workers, Their Roles and Tasks*. London: National Institute of Social Work, Bedford Square Press (Barclay Report).

Bebbington, A. and Miles, J. (1988) *Children Entering Care: a Need Indicator for In Care Services for Children*. Canterbury: PSSRU, University of Kent.

Benzeval, M. and Judge, K. (1992) 'Deprivation and poor health in childhood: prospects for prevention', in H. Otto and G. Flosser (eds), *How to Organise Prevention – Political, Professional and Organisational Challenges to Social Services*. Berlin: Walter de Gruyter.

Berridge, D. (1985) *Children's Homes*. Oxford: Basil Blackwell.

Brayne, H. and Martin, G. (1990) *Law for Social Workers*. London: Blackstone.

Brazil, E. and Steward, S. (1992) 'My own flesh and blood', *Community Care*, 12 April: 12–13.

Cox, A., Pound, A. and Puckering, C. (1992) 'NEWPIN: a befriending scheme and therapeutic network for carers of young children', in J. Gibbons (ed.), *The Children Act 1989 and Family Support*. London: HMSO. pp. 37–49.

Dale, P., Davies, M., Morrison, T. and Waters, J. (1986) *Dangerous Families: Assessment and Treatment of Child Abuse.* London: Tavistock.

Department of Health (1982) *Child Abuse: A Study of Inquiry Reports.* London: HMSO.

Department of Health (1990) *The Care of Children. Principles and Practice in Regulations and Guidance.* London: HMSO.

Department of Health (1991a) *Child Abuse: A Study of Inquiry Reports 1980–1989.* London: HMSO.

Department of Health (1991b) *Patterns and Outcomes in Child Placement. Messages from Current Research and their Implications.* London: HMSO.

Department of Health (1991c) *Working Together under the Children Act 1989. A Guide to Arrangements for Inter-agency Co-operation for the Protection of Children from Abuse.* London: HMSO.

Department of Health (1991d) *The Children Act 1989 Guidance and Regulations: Volume 2: Family Support, Day Care and Educational Provisions.* London: HMSO.

Department of Health (1991e) *The Children Act 1989 Guidance and Regulations: Volume 4: Residential Care.* London: HMSO.

Department of Health (1993) *Health and Personal Social Services Statistics for England.* London: Government Statistical Service.

Department of Health (1995) *Child Protection: Messages from Research.* London: HMSO.

DHSS (1988) *Report of the Inquiry into Child Abuse in Cleveland 1987: Short Version Extracted from the Complete Text.* London: HMSO.

Farmer, E. and Owen, M. (1993) *Decision Making, Intervention and Outcome in Child Protection Work.* Bristol: University of Bristol Press.

Franklin, B. and Parton, N. (eds) (1991) *Social Work, the Media and Public Relations.* London: Routledge.

Furniss, T. (1991) *Multi-professional Handbook of Child Sexual Abuse. Integrated Management, Therapy, and Legal Interventions.* London: Routledge.

Gibbons, J. (1991) 'Children in need and their families: outcomes of referrals to social services', *British Journal of Social Work*, 21(3): 217–28.

Gibbons, J. (ed.) (1992) *The Children Act 1989 and Family Support: Principles into Practice.* London: HMSO.

Gibbons, J., Conroy, S. and Bell, C. (1993) *Operation of Child Protection Registers.* Norwich: University of East Anglia Press.

Giller, H. (1993) *Children in Need: Definition, Management and Monitoring.* London: Department of Health.

Glaser, D. and Frosh, S. (1988) *Child Sexual Abuse.* Harlow: Longman.

Hardiker, P. (1992) 'Family support services and children with disabilities', in J. Gibbons (ed.), *The Children Act and Family Support: Principles into Practice.* London: HMSO.

Holman, B. (1988) *Putting Families First: Prevention and Child Care.* London: Macmillan.

Holman, B. (1989) 'Family centres', in S. Morgan and P. Reighton (eds), *Child Care: Concerns and Conflicts.* London: Hodder & Stoughton. pp. 155–67.

Jackson, S. (1989) 'Education of children in care', in B. Kahan (ed.), *Child Care. Research, Policy and Practice.* Sevenoaks: Hodder & Stoughton. pp. 133–51.

Jordan, B. (1984) *Invitation to Social Work.* Oxford: Martin Robertson.

Little, M. and Gibbons, J. (1993) 'Predicting the rate of children on the child protection register', *Research, Policy and Planning*, 10: 15–18.

Marsh, P. and Fisher, M. (1992) *Good Intentions: Developing Partnership in Social Services*. York: Joseph Rowntree Foundation.

Millham, S., Bullock, R., Hosie, K. and Little, M. (1986) *Lost in Care: The Problems of Maintaining Links between Children in Care and their Families*. Aldershot: Gower.

Mitchell, G. (1989) 'Professional decision-making in child abuse cases: the social worker's dilemma', *Child Abuse Review*, 3(1): 7–12.

National Foster Care Association [NFCA] (1992) *Foster Care Finance: Advice and Information on the Cost of Caring for a Child*. London: NFCA.

Packman, J., Randell, J. and Jacques, N. (1986) *Who Needs Care?* Oxford: Blackwell.

Parton, N. (1985) *The Politics of Child Abuse*. Basingstoke: Macmillan.

Parton, N. (1986) 'The Beckford Report: a critical appraisal', *British Journal of Social Work*, 16(5): 511–30.

Preston-Shoot, M. and Agass, D. (1990) *Making Sense of Social Work: Psychodynamics, Systems and Practice*. Basingstoke: Macmillan.

Prosser, P. (1978) *Perspectives in Foster Care*. Windsor: NFER.

Prosser, P. (1992) *Child Abuse Investigations: The Families' Perspective*. Oxford: Parents Against Injustice.

Robinson, M. (1978) *Schools and Social Work*. London: Routledge & Kegan Paul.

Rose, W. (1993) 'Foreword', in J. Gibbons (ed.), *The Children Act 1989 and Family Support: Principles into Practice*. London: HMSO. pp. ix–xiii.

Rowe, J. Hundleby, M. and Garnett, L. (1989) *Child Care Now*. London: British Agencies for Adoption and Fostering.

Ruddock, M. (1991) 'A receptacle for public anger', in B. Franklin and N. Parton (eds), *Social Work, the Media and Public Relations*. London: Routledge. pp. 107–16.

Smith, M. and Bentovim, A. (1994) 'Sexual abuse', in M. Rutter, E. Taylor and L. Hersov (eds), *Child and Adolescent Psychiatry: Modern Approaches*, 3rd edn. Oxford: Blackwell Scientific Publications.

Social Services Inspectorate (1993) *Evaluating Performance in Child Protection: A Framework for the Inspection of Local Authority Social Services Practice and Systems*. London: HMSO.

Taylor, S. (1989) 'How prevalent is it?', in W. Stainton Rogers, D. Hevey and E. Ash (eds), *Child Abuse and Neglect: Facing the Challenge*. London: Batsford. pp. 40–49.

Thoburn, J., Lewis, A. and Shemmings, D. (1993) *Family Participation in Child Protection*. Norwich: University of East Anglia Press.

Tunstill, J. (1992) 'Local authority policies on children in need', in J. Gibbons (ed.), *The Children Act 1989 and Family Support: Principles into Practice*. London: HMSO. pp. 155–66.

Ward, D. and Mullender, A. (1991) 'Empowerment and oppression: an indissoluble pairing for contemporary social work', *Critical Social Policy*, 32: 21–30.

# 5

# Community Care and Social Work with Adults

This chapter covers the concept of work with 'adults' and the historical context of discrimination against them; the background to community care and the role of social work within this. It considers the effects of the discordant blends of knowledge and skills brought to this area of work, and care management as a needs-led process of assessment and planning. At the same time, user involvement is explored within the context of 'partnership' as a means of working towards empowering users (issues relating to liberty and protection); and the disability movement's view of community care is also discussed. Following from that, some of the general skills and knowledge needed for work with 'adults' are referred to, and the role of the approved social worker and the appropriate interview in relation to work with people in mental distress is discussed as a 'blueprint' for all work with 'adults'. Finally, efforts to offer alternatives to compulsion under the law for people experiencing mental distress are covered and issues relating to 'adult'/elder abuse are critically examined.

## The historical context of discrimination and the concept of work with 'adults'

While the legal definition of 'adult' varies from 16 to 21 years depending on the issue under consideration, many people can be regarded as an adult in law, without being afforded the privilege of being treated as one.

Adults with learning and physical disabilities, mental distress and older people frequently are regarded or treated as children; are denied the ability to take control of their own lives; are excluded from major decision-making processes on an individual, institutional and structural level; infantilised by a society which often sees and treats them as being in need of protection, yet denies them equal access to education, employment, leisure and so on.

While different societies and cultures have differing attitudes to mental health, disability and age, examples of discrimination can be found in all parts of the world and over many centuries (see, for instance, Morris, 1991). In Britain this is evidenced by the abuses experienced by many of those housed in the original asylums, large hospitals, workhouses and other institutions which were still in widespread use earlier this century (Goffman, 1961; Morris, 1991). The offensive language in popular use relating to disability, mental distress and ageing, often based on negative assumptions and stereotypes, points to the powerful and deeply entrenched nature of this continuing discrimination.

There are various theoretical explanations relating to the source of this discrimination (Davies, 1982; Fanon, 1967; Morris, 1991; Tinker, 1984). The denial of basic human rights to people who through ignorance or prejudice are perceived and stereotyped as 'different' or 'dangerous' is familiar in relation to discrimination applied to other minority groups. The value judgements brought to bear on these differences are the problem: racism, sexism, disablism, homo-hatred, ageism and classism are all prime examples of this, and when combinations of these discriminations are operating together, individuals' experience of oppression is compounded. Adult experiences may include illness, disability, mental distress, poverty, or other forms of oppression mentioned above. Any or all of these may be relevant at that time to our involvement as social workers (Morris, 1991).

Although pockets of good practice have always existed, it seems likely that the level of discrimination and lack of value society attaches to adults in need of support is reflected in, and accounts for, generally poor practice in this area.

Research indicates that work with adults attracts fewer qualified social workers, who receive lower status, lower pay and are likely to receive less training than their peers (Oliver, 1993; Tinker, 1984). The 'canteen culture' of social work itself offers the unstated, and sometimes stated, view that 'real' social work happens with children and families, and that anyone choosing to work with adults (with the possible exception of mental health) does so because they are somewhat lacking in skills. Conversely, if workers are perceived to be skilled and competent, if they are working with adults the implication is that this is a waste of training and expertise. However, the major recent changes in legislation (e.g. the National Health Service and Community Care Act 1990) have led to changes in work with adults, and will hopefully lead to changes in overall attitudes.

Work with adults can be seen as a de-stigmatising process which brings together the areas of disability, mental health and ageing. When we refer to people as 'adults in need of support' rather than people who are learning or physically disabled, mentally ill or ageing, we begin from the principle that they are individuals in their own right. Acknowledging people's ability and right to define themselves as they choose is fundamental to respecting them as individuals. Similarly, given that language is dynamic, holding different meanings for different people in different contexts, listening, seeking agreement and shared understanding is central to setting the tone and expectation of working *alongside* people.

Since local authorities cannot provide services without statutory requirement, we need to be clear about to whom the legislation applies. However, categorising individuals in relation to their disability or age can have negative and damaging consequences. Local authorities attempting to offer a more focused service through specialist divisions run the risk of compounding this labelling process, and knowledge of the power of labels and the consequent effect on normal social relationships is essential (see, for instance, Becker, 1963; Downes and Rock, 1988; Smith, 1995; Laing, 1967).

An understanding of anti-oppressive and anti-discriminatory ways of working, a commitment to social justice and social welfare to enhance the quality of people's lives and to repudiate all forms of negative discrimination is essential (CCETSW, 1991, 1995). Valuing individuals' rights to dignity, respect, privacy, confidentiality, choice and protection from abuse and exploitation is also integral to the aims of community care.

### The background to community care

Since the 1950s there have been various attempts by successive governments towards community care. This was due to numerous factors, including exposure of abuse in all areas of care for adults; economic considerations; developments in pharmacology; and an increasing understanding of the impacts of institutionalisation.

The National Assistance Act 1948, and the Chronically Sick and Disabled Persons Act 1970 (CSDPA) arising from the Seebohm Report (Department of Health and Social Security, 1968) were the main legislative influences relating to social work with adults. These concentrated on the local authority's duty to assess and provide those eligible with services. Oliver (1993:129) argues that Seebohm did not create generic departments but specialist childcare ones, where the needs of children were met by trained professionals and other needs and obligations were met by unqualified staff, welfare assistants and the like.

Fourteen years later the Barclay Committee (Barclay, 1982) discovered that children and families work was proportionately allocated more to senior and qualified social workers, while unqualified, inexperienced or assistant social workers took on the work with adults (Oliver, 1993). Work with adults often tended to be of a crisis intervention nature, that is to say when an elderly person, previously offered little or no support, was in need of residential care and was considered to be at crisis point. Social workers have consistently been criticised for the inadequate service they offer to adults. Oliver (1993:14) writes thus:

> Social workers' failure to develop an adequate theoretical and practical base for their interventions has led to criticisms, notably by disabled people themselves, who have accused social workers of ignorance about handicapping conditions, benefits and rights, failing to recognise the need for practical assistance as well as verbal advice and to involve disabled people in the training process.

Local authorities have always produced their own policies and procedures in an attempt to offer consistent standards of work to meet their statutory duties. However, the piecemeal historical development of the law relating to adults has not given this area of social work the overall structure it needs.

Although there has been development of policy and good practice in some areas, other areas of work, for instance that relating to sexuality and sexual identity, have often been ignored or tabooed in social work, particularly in work with adults with learning disabilities. Ageism, disablism, sexism and homo-hatred all have played their role in enabling the denial or avoidance of these issues; and if adults are regarded as having a sexual identity at all, it is generally assumed to be heterosexual.

The National Health Service and Community Care Act 1990 introduced major changes to the way health and social services work with adults, and to the organisational, philosophical and funding structures underpinning the delivery of services to those who need them. In addition, the government's expectations regarding this law's implementation have been backed by serious financial penalties if local authorities do not comply.

### Community care

The law relating to adults has developed in a 'higgledy piggledy way, producing overlaps between legislation' (Fishwick, 1992:103). However, the National Health Service and Community Care Act 1990 and its guidelines largely encapsulate the government's approach towards adults in need of support. The government's position is well presented in the Department of Health's *Caring for People* (1989:101):

> Many people need some extra help and support at some stage in their lives as a result of illness or temporary disability. Some people as a result

of the effects of old age, of mental illness including dementia, of mental handicap or physical disability or sensory impairment, have continuing need for care on a longer term basis. People with drug and alcohol related disorders, people with multiple handicaps and people with progressive illnesses such as A.I.D.S or multiple sclerosis may also need community care at some time.

Community care's main aims are to enable people to live as independently, and for as long as possible, in the community with maximum control and choice over their lives. This is to be provided through a range of flexible services, which respond, with minimum intrusion, to those individuals and their carers who are in most need.

The development of a range of independent sector support services alongside good-quality public resources, which offer tax-payers choice and better value for money, are key objectives (Department of Health, 1989). While this has led to the creation of many innovative services, without effective mechanisms to collate and distribute this information they are likely to remain as local initiatives only.

Agencies are to be clearly accountable for their performance. Local authorities have duties to publish community care plans and information about services, eligibility criteria and complaints procedures. At the same time they are to establish registration and inspection units for their own and independent sector residential units and to consult with service users, their carers and the community, regarding their needs.

Many might argue community care merely formalises what was previously good practice, though that may have been the exception rather than the rule. Community care does offer a clear, legally binding and consistent framework, which attempts to standardise the approach to work with adults. Nevertheless, there are many inconsistencies in the law's implementation, and it has been criticised for its loose, flexible requirements compared with those of the Children Act 1989 (Haslett, 1991). Practice and service standards vary, compounded by local authorities' differing budgetary constraints, which potentially affect staffing levels, the quality of assessments, user choice and the levels of eligibility criteria in operation.

Scepticism is common regarding the 'real', as opposed to the political, agenda of community care as a cheap option, inadequately funded and placing the onus on informal carers – families, friends, neighbours and particularly women (Finch and Groves, 1983). Indeed, this political agenda – which exploits the ideological desirability of community care but starves community agencies and providers of adequate resources – has been the main and most consistent focus of criticism of the policy. See, for example, the main concerns of the Griffiths Report (Griffiths, 1988). Consequently, front-line staff are placed in the position of refusing services to those in need, which runs counter to the values of social work.

Stevenson and Parsloe (1993:6) highlight some of the ideological confusions of community care, including the expectation that families care for their own as well as their neighbours; the message from the government to the independent sector to create wealth yet provide voluntary services; the notion to free citizens from interference by the state, yet that vulnerable adults must be protected; the importance that users have choice, yet must have their needs assessed by the local authority: carers' and users' needs are to be assessed, yet the possibility of conflict between those needs is rarely addressed in the accompanying guidance relating to community care.

Stevenson and Parsloe (1993:32) also suggest that local administrative procedures could deny the proper fulfilment of the assessment process to the detriment of both workers and users. They argue that bureaucratic over-regulation could jeopardise effective application of legislation and ultimately lead to disempowerment of workers and users.

But more serious than that, there is evidence to suggest that social work agencies and practitioners are still struggling to come to terms with the implementation of the Act. For example Smale et al. (1993:2) point out the pressing ideological and practical tasks currently facing social work, arguing that:

> To empower users, carers and the older people they work with and to respond to the unique circumstances that confront them on a day to day basis, professionals have to reinvent their practice and their perception of particular problems and solutions they find themselves in.

A distinction between the roles of purchasers and paid providers of care is also central to the philosophy of objective assessments of need. Care management is envisaged as a 'brokerage' role, selecting the best from a range of services to meet the individuals' needs most appropriately. However, the Department of Health and Social Services Inspectorate (SSI) does not preclude care managers from undertaking direct work with users to meet an identified need. As a result some local authorities have chosen to interpret care management and social work separately while others incorporate those tasks into the care management role.

## Social work as a direct service provider

Many local authorities responded to the demands of community care and the Children Act 1989 by reorganising from generic to specialist divisions.

As suggested elsewhere (cf. Smale et al., 1993; Vass and Taylor, 1995) social workers' experience of this process has been quite difficult if not dramatic. One of the hardest transitions for social workers working with adults to make is that from of 'doing social work' to 'doing care management'. Many workers and service users are unclear about the differences involved and the confusion is compounded by the difficulty experienced at management level as to which direction to follow and how that direction may be adequately financed. Workers find this experience de-skilling, fearing that the expertise they needed as social workers will not be used in a short-term purchasing role and will be lost. They feel that the number and pressure of referrals to teams, which are far more than originally envisaged, will lead towards a conveyor-belt style of working and will affect the quality of service offered.

Many fear the care management role will preclude opportunities for longer-term work with people, from which they feel they had previously gained job satisfaction. However, it has become evident that, where an individual's needs are complex and frequently changing, care management will involve longer-term intervention. Care management can involve co-working, individually allocated, and duty and crisis intervention work, while regular reviews offer an opportunity for a consistent and continuing role for social workers.

Care management is a complex and demanding area of work for which the skills, knowledge and value base of social work are ideally suited, as Chapter 2 on values has cogently argued. In the role of care manager, the social worker is to purchase and arrange appropriate services to meet assessed needs. The care plan might involve family work, counselling and so forth, which may or may not be provided by the care manager. Where there is no provision for the social work task to be undertaken separately many care managers may find themselves having to incorporate this into their work.

The role of social work as a direct provider is indispensable if it is to offer the full range of resources to adults to meet their needs adequately. This can and will be provided in a range of settings including residential, group living, day care, community, hospital and fieldwork, and can be achieved through multi-disciplinary or central social work teams, or bought in from specialist independent sector organisations. This last option, which is the least used so far, could arguably be the most appropriate for the future direction of social work with adults, as it is more likely to be able to provide a flexible and empowering service. Organisations set up and run by service users themselves have an essential contribution and role in relation to needs-led assessment and care planning. Some organisations have also produced their own guidance for good practice in relation to community care (see for instance Centre for Policy on Ageing, 1990).

### Discordant blends of knowledge, skills and values involved in social work with adults

The National Health Service and Community Care Act 1990 outlines the approach both the health and social services must take to working with adults in need of support and services (Department of Health, 1989). The rationale behind joining together these disciplines is to create an opportunity to streamline services, avoid duplication of roles and create a more flexible, efficient and 'seamless' service for users.

Housing, education, leisure, benefits agencies, the police, voluntary, private and community organisations and networks have key roles to play, and need to adopt a coherent and cooperative way of working together to ensure that community care achieves its stated goals. Of course, this inter-agency aspect is not without problems. It is often difficult for diverse agencies to co-work due to severe rifts in ideologies and missions, as well as because they are all competing in the economy for resources (see, for example, Smith, 1995: ch.5; Vass 1990:73–6; May and Vass, 1996: ch. 10).

Notwithstanding these difficulties, workers will need to be able to 'manage the involvement, contribution, co-operation and partnership between the Local Authority and other authorities and professionals involved in providing services' (Department of Health, 1989:19). The government's view is that a range of professionals including social workers, home care organisers and community nurses (because of their regular contact with users) will be particularly suited to care management (Department of Health, 1989). This brings together very different knowledge, skills and value bases from health and social services approaches. Since the experience and training undertaken by nurses, social workers and home care workers varies tremendously, inter-agency work will be lacking in some areas for some workers, and an ability to transfer appropriate knowledge and skills to new situations will be essential.

A multi-disciplinary, inter-agency approach offers a wealth of shared knowledge, skills and expertise but can present difficulties of an organisational and operational type (Department of Health,

1991a, 1991b). Clear strategic planning by local and health authorities is needed and workers must be able to operate effectively within these structures. 'Locality meetings', where workers link and meet regularly with local clinics, general practitioners' surgeries or other local community resources, offer examples of how good liaison and shared understanding towards a more efficient and seamless service can be established.

The government acknowledges the need for the training and retraining of all staff involved in community care in order to standardise the quality of practice and services. The new Diploma in Social Work (CCETSW, 1991, 1995) and National Vocational Qualification (NVQ) initiatives for social care staff are a case in point. However, there has been much debate about whether some NVQs go far enough in preparing workers adequately for the work they will be undertaking.

Given the range of skills, knowledge and values brought to work with adults it is even more essential that there are agreed competences for this work, though the real danger here is that competences can become, if not checked, as we have argued in the introduction and final chapter in this volume, convenient 'shopping lists' which are equally and conveniently ticked off without the workers demonstrating any clear intellectual and practical skills in delivering services.

### Care management as a needs-led process of assessment and care-planning

Community care legislation focuses on the principle of a needs-led rather than a service-led response to work with adults. Assessment is that of an individual's needs, and care management is the process of tailoring services to individual needs.

The Department of Health outlines seven 'core tasks' to clearly structure the process of care management: this constitutes a major step towards an agreed approach and competence in work with adults:

- publishing information about the assistance which is available for certain needs;
- determining the level of assessment by making an initial identification of need and matching it to the appropriate level of assessment;
- assessing need, relating this to agency policies and priorities, agreeing the objectives identified, and incorporating these into a 'care plan';

- implementing the care plan by securing the necessary services or resources;
- monitoring by the continuous support and control of the implementation of the care plan;
- reviewing by reassessing the needs and outcomes of the services with a view to revising the care plan, if appropriate, at specified intervals. (Department of Health, 1991b:11–12).

There are difficulties relating to how far it is possible to achieve a truly needs-led assessment and care planning process, as well as serious criticism of the factors limiting its realisation.

A fundamental conflict exists between community care's aim to promote independence and individuals' control over their own lives on the one hand, and the maintenance of assessment, definition of needs and access to services under local authority control or direction on the other (Morris, 1993; Oliver, 1993; Stevenson and Parsloe, 1993).

Arguably, the only truly needs-led process would be that of users identifying their own needs, and being given cash to meet these as they wish (Morris, 1993; Oliver, 1993), though even this model assumes that all people are rational or capable of making the right choices. While viewing self-assessment as an ideal, there is concern that given finite resources this would lead to unrealistic expectations, resulting in local authorities being taken to court over unmet need, with the most powerful users getting the most resources. How real needs-led provision of services can be against the existing background of budgetary, resource and organisational constraints is a matter of conjecture. Nonetheless, while in the longer term this is a civil rights issue, given the parameters, we can try to work towards making the assessment and care planning process as empowering as possible.

It is essential to separate the process of assessment of need from that of service planning to meet those needs. This is particularly difficult, if not impossible, when the worker undertaking the assessment also holds the budget for services. Yet separating the two roles to aid a more objective assessment raises different issues in relation to the numbers of workers, intrusion and continuity involved for the user.

The ability to facilitate people in identifying their own needs, wants and choices, is particularly important if people have been denied or discouraged from this in the past. If users have previously experienced discrimination or negative responses from workers, they may have very low expectations or fear losing what services they do receive, if they make too many demands (Morris, 1993).

People may request a service, for instance a day centre, because that is their experience or knowledge of what social services traditionally provide, not necessarily because that is the service they need. Users should be enabled to explore what it is about that service they feel comfortable with or require, and be given the relevant information they need to make informed decisions.

While we must respect a person's right not to explore this further, in certain situations this right may have to be balanced against their own or others' well-being and safety and in relation to the agencies' legal responsibilities. Sensitively overcoming barriers to clear communication, which may include issues around language, learning, speech, culture, gender, class and so forth, is essential to working in partnership in an empowering way (Smale et al., 1993). Workers will need to consider if they are the most appropriate people to undertake the work, and whether an independent advocate, or other person close to the user is needed. Good interpersonal, engagement and counselling skills (Egan, 1986) and the ability to build trusting relationships quickly are important.

Gathering and evaluating information relevant to an holistic assessment of needs must take account of an individual within the unique context of their complete life experience. In addition to those areas already mentioned this should include their family, community or other support networks; education; employment; leisure; physical and mental well-being; housing; and financial situation.

A client-centred approach, informed by anti-discriminatory practice, and an awareness of the possible pressures, differing agendas and needs of those involved, and of the impact these may have on the user themselves, is essential. An obvious example might be a request to place an older person in a home for their own safety.

Workers need to be aware of, and sensitive to, the role, involvement, stresses and separate needs of those close to the user. Whilst an individual may be in the role of carer this may not be through choice but through lack of alternatives and may not be appropriate. Users and their carers may have conflicting needs, views or wishes, and workers must be able to use the basic knowledge and skills referred to in previous chapters in order to work sensitively and competently in this area. It may also be appropriate to offer a carer an assessment in their own right which might best be undertaken by another worker, or indeed another agency.

A needs-led care-planning process must take account of the individual requirements of a person in relation to the service provided. For example, someone needing assistance to wash and dress in the mornings should be helped to identify how and by whom that service should be provided. It may not be possible to meet these needs precisely because the service is unavailable or the eligibility criteria exclude the person, or there is no budget available, and workers must be aware of their agencies' policies and criteria relating to access to services, the identification and recording of 'unmet need', and its political and legal implications. This, and a good knowledge of existing resources, offers workers a key role in identifying gaps in provision, and in its future planning and development.

An innovative approach to negotiating, planning and arranging flexible, cost-effective services is essential. Skills required for needs-led service planning include budgeting, contracting and service specification; quality assurance and control; and an understanding of the factors and impact of economic, political, racial, social and cultural issues in the context of service delivery.

Users may be limited in their opportunities to monitor or feed back any difficulties relating to their care plan, and may not be able to rely on anyone else to do this for them – for instance when a person is confused or has short-term memory loss. A range of working methods may be useful here, including the involvement of those close to the person; the use of advocates; 'spot' visits and telephone calls; and mechanisms to record visits or contact by those involved. These methods, underpinned by an awareness of confidentiality issues, and a sensitivity towards the user's right to privacy, should always be founded on clear agreements between the user and all those involved.

### User involvement and the concept of partnership and empowerment

The central principle of community care is that if assessment, care management and services are to meet the needs of adults using them, then users must be fully involved and consulted, throughout the process, both on an individual and on a strategic planning level (Donlan, 1993).

Workers have an important role in supporting and being involved in user forums and regular community-based meetings; they have a responsibility to promote good working links with voluntary and user-led organisations, advocacy initiatives and carer centres. The gist of all this is to enable users to participate fully and give regular feedback. Working in partnership with users is essential towards this end and community social work approaches encapsulate many useful ways of working in this area.

Whilst people now have right of access to their files, a more proactive approach, for instance recording information with and in front of users, would be helpful in demystifying the process and allowing users to 'own' the content. An open and honest approach, particularly when people may be suspicious or fearful of social work intentions or motives, combined with an awareness of the possible communication needs of service users, is important.

But involving users goes beyond mere contact and openness. The relationship should also be at a practical level whereby users are encouraged and enabled to be involved in securing appropriate resources: for instance in drawing up job descriptions and interviewing their own personal assistants; and in defining the standards and measures of the success of those services secured, so that they can actively contribute their views and criticisms. What this means is that the review process must be responsive to the dynamic nature of people's lives and its effectiveness will relate directly to the quality and level of involvement of the users in the assessment, care-planning and monitoring process. Indeed, it has to be emphasised that within community care local authorities are perceived as *enablers*, delivering services in conjunction *with* people rather than *to* them, which is the essence of the partnership relationship.

Despite that partnership relationship and the goal of achieving it, partnerships will always involve power differentials. It is important to be realistic and to acknowledge the barriers to a truly equal partnership with users, and to explore as well as, in many instances, accept the power service purchasers and providers have in legislative, organisational and social terms. As Wertheimer (1993:13) puts it:

> power is something you recognise when you haven't got it. I suspect most users have a very vivid sense of what it is like to lack power. I suggest that it's something which people working in services tend not even to think about. . . . Its existence is demonstrated when people feel it's unsafe to criticise services because they might lose the support they get, however unsatisfactory that is. Power is inherent in the fact that services often do things to or for people, not with them. Maybe this is something individual staff need to address for themselves? Where and in what ways do I exercise power over people?

Working in partnership involves at some crucial stage negotiating and redistributing power if that partnership is indeed a working relationship. That means, at some stage, giving up an 'all encompassing expert role' (Smale et al., 1993) and making efforts to allow users to define and promote their own understanding, views and action plans in consideration. *In toto*, workers must actively share thoughts and ideas and listen to others' points of view rather than just do as they themselves define a situation or simply as they feel expected to do (Stevenson and Parsloe, 1993).

Assessments which are undertaken as a one-way process of information gathering by the worker are disempowering for users and often may result in a superficial and oversimplistic identification of their needs. Smale et al. (1993) highlight the benefits of work with users which involves an exchange of information, sharing perceptions of situations, problems and solutions and which offers a more empowering approach. Similarly, in service provision, providing support to enable users to do their own shopping, for example, is likely to empower them more than arranging for this to be done for them.

Iveson's (1990) work with older people and their families suggests that a good basis for empowering practice with all adults is a client-centred and anti-discriminatory approach which assumes older people have a responsible and actively influential role in the relationships and situations in which they are involved and are able to exercise choices. He notes that 'There is no way of knowing that all people retain the capacity to choose, but believing that they do leads to one sort of behaviour and believing that they don't leads to another' (Iveson, 1990:15).

Many of the adults with whom social workers work will have a common experience of disempowerment, given that they often experience discrimination and oppression. Working in ways that attempt to empower users as far as possible is key in trying to redress this. Stevenson and Parsloe (1993:4) have noted that 'Whilst equality is not synonymous with empowerment, they are profoundly connected.' Having said that, it is important to acknowledge that the relationship between equality and empowerment is a very complicated one and that the concept of 'power' or 'empowerment' can be very elusive and may mean different things to different people. There is a fundamental conflict between independence and protection, empowerment and individual choice.

Social workers' powers derive from statute, and while the values that underpin their work are indeed those of maximising individuals' empowerment, independence and control over their own lives social workers are also, as Fishwick (1992:8) points out: 'the means by which society manages deviance from what are assumed to be agreed norms of behaviour. Such professionals find themselves, therefore, with caring and controlling functions, and constantly operating between individuals' needs and society's needs.' Given the range of powers by which people's liberty can be restricted or removed, it is essential that workers use these constructively, and are able to protect users' rights where necessary. Clarity regarding what is meant by 'protection', whose protection we are considering and why, is vital.

Assessment of risk and risk taking is central to any discussion involving independence, liberty and protection, and have been more readily associated with child protection. Certainly, there are few policy guidelines relating to issues of risk in work with adults, and this is an area needing further attention.

### Radical critique by the disability movement

Many disability groups, whilst welcoming the majority of the aims and principles of the community care legislation, remain highly critical of certain fundamental ideological conflicts they see at its core, which give them cause to question how realistically achievable and implementable those aims and principles may be. Central to these concerns is the concept and understanding of 'independent living' and what is understood by 'independence'. This, rather than being associated, as it traditionally is, with an individual's ability to be self-reliant and self-supporting, should be seen as individuals having control over all aspects of their lives, and as an issue of civil rights. Morris (1993:38) argues thus:

> The aim of independent living is held back by an ideology at the heart of community care policies, which does not recognise the civil rights of disabled people but instead considers them to be dependent people and in need of care. Associated with this is the central importance given to the role of 'informal carers' – partners, relatives and friends of 'dependent people' whose unpaid assistance is seen as vital in keeping down the costs of community care policies.

Indeed, the government's stated intention that informal carers have a key role to play in community care rests on the assumption that informal caring networks exist and have an independent life of their own. This is an assumption which has been questioned and criticised (see, for instance, Finch and Groves, 1980). There is also an assumption that there is a willingness and choice on behalf of carers to care, and on behalf of users to be cared for, in this way. Such an understanding of informal networks does not take account of the possible effects and consequences upon those relationships. As Morris (1993:10) puts it:

> Are they [disabled people] merely 'dependants' of long-suffering carers? Do they have nothing to offer a relationship other than a 'burden of caring'? And what is it like to receive care from those you love? What effect does it have on your relationships? How does it compare with receiving assistance from those who are paid to give it?

Yet, if informal carers and users have no alternatives in relation to the caring role which, given the criticisms levelled at community care in relation to inadequate funding and resourcing, may well be the case, there is indeed a conflict of ideology present, since choice is a cornerstone principle of the policy.

Morris (1993) argues further that the concept of independence as meaning the ability to have control and choice over all aspects of an individual's life applies to all adults. Whilst this is a valid point, it is also important to recognise that the degree of choice individuals are able to exercise in their lives varies. Social workers often work with extremely vulnerable individuals and it is essential that they acknowledge and undertake their responsibilities here sensitively and appropriately.

It is worth noting that the Disability Rights Bill (Ogden, 1994; George and Lineham, 1994), which would have enshrined and protected many civil rights for disabled people in legislation and empowered them considerably, was recently blocked by the government on the grounds that it would be too costly to implement. This offers a powerful example of how political and economic contingency appears to override the socially desirable value of empowering a section of the population who have been seen and defined as the 'dependent'. Furthermore, the government's action violated the very spirit of their own, already enacted, legislation – the National Health Service and Community Care Act 1990.

It would appear that it is easier to sound the trumpet call for community care and empowerment than it is to put it into practice, as there may be other ideological, sociopolitical and economic forces at play.

Social workers have been justly criticised for the limited approaches they have often employed in work with adults. Oliver (1993) argues that, all too often, approaches to work with disabled people have focused on either a diagnosis (which concentrates too narrowly on the physical and medical factors relating to an individual's disability), or an assumptive judgement that to be disabled is a tragedy requiring an adjustment on behalf of the disabled person, and which generally assumes the need for bereavement counselling intervention. Instead, Oliver calls for an anti-discriminatory and non-pathologising approach which moves the focus away from the physical limitations of individuals and on to the physical and social environments which impose limitations upon certain groups or categories of people.

Some of Oliver's criticisms are valid, given that employing any one of the above models to the exclusion of other approaches is unhelpful and oversimplifies the complexity of individuals' experiences. However, it would be a mistake to totally reject the potential relevance or value that these models may have within an eclectic approach to working with adults. While an understanding and awareness of different approaches is essential, the important point is the need to approach each individual's situation and needs as unique to them. Rather than entering into a working relationship with a user with a preconceived 'repair kit of theory' that may well have no relevance whatsoever to their situation, which, in fact, may well not be in need of repair, the worker must retain an open mind and be willing to redefine and reconstruct the situation according to the individual context of each user.

## What do we need to know in order to work competently with adults?

The diverse range of skills, knowledge and approaches of social work are all relevant and needed in work with adults, and some of those which are generally and more specifically applicable are covered in this section.

Adults are amongst the poorest and most poorly housed members of society (Hicks, 1988; Rowlings, 1981). This means that workers must have a good knowledge of welfare and housing rights and legislation, or of where to find this information.

Some broad socio-medical and socio-psychological knowledge can minimise unnecessary intrusion into people's lives in relation to sensitive and personal issues, although we should not make assumptions, and having an idea of how an illness and disability may progress may enable us to assist users in planning for possible changes. This does not mean that social workers should assume the role of expert in a field in which they are not experts.

A problem-solving approach, focusing on working in partnership with users to empower them as far as possible, can usefully draw on psychodynamic, task-centred, behavioural and social learning theories.

Thinking as we often do of adults and their carers, rather than adults and their families, we may overlook the need or use of family work (Iveson, 1990). The application of systems theory can inform work with a person in relation to their family, wider community networks or others with whom they are involved, including those residing in group living settings. Group-work theories and methods can also be applied to family, community and individual work approaches. However, it is important that we see theories as a means of making sense of our actions and do not confuse them with reality (Iveson, 1990).

Knowledge of human development and the life cycle, which focuses on key times of change or stress, is important, but caution must be exercised as these theories have limitations, based as they often are upon discriminating assumptions. For example, Erikson's (1982) 'stages of development', covering detailed life changes up to 'adulthood', jumps from retirement to death, assuming a period of up to fifty years involves little or no significant development or change.

In order to work with older people, theories relating to the later life cycle, ageing process, reminiscence and reality orientation work can be useful. However, the assertion that ours is the reality to which someone must conform is not always helpful, and social workers should beware of colluding with ageist assumptions by using this as a process focusing purely on past experiences and points of reference, rather than on a person's present value and future life. Life-history work may offer a more positive approach here.

Finally, workers need to understand their own roles and responsibilities and those of agencies, in order to offer or refer people to the most appropriate service.

## The role of the approved social worker

In working with people in mental distress, local authorities have the duty to provide sufficient numbers of approved social workers (ASWs) to carry out their responsibilities under the Mental Health Act 1983 (section 114). They must be appropriately trained and competent to work with, and assess the needs of people 'who are suffering with a mental disorder' (Fishwick, 1992). The guidance for good practice and the implementation of the Act is contained in the *Mental Health Act Code of Practice* (Department of Health and Welsh Office, 1990).

ASWs have considerable powers under the Act, most notably their personal responsibilities relating to making applications for compulsory admissions to hospital. Knowledge and understanding of the relevant law, guidance and policies are needed. Ensuring that users are aware of their rights, and are empowered to make use of them, is important, particularly in relation to compulsory admission and the role and powers of the Mental Health Review Tribunal and Mental Health Act Commission (Department of Health and Welsh Office, 1990).

The introduction of ASWs could be seen as requiring an increase in the range of social workers' knowledge and skills, leading to higher standards of assessment and training. It was arguably 'the first statutorily required specialism since Seebohm' (Brown, 1987:17). The 'ASW model' can be effectively transferred and used in other areas of work with adults, particularly given the absence of specific practice guidance elsewhere, other than that relating to the process of care management (Department of Health, 1991a; 1991b).

The principles underpinning work with people in mental distress highlight the importance of individual, holistic, needs-led assessments and are as follows:

1. respecting, and considering users' individual qualities and diversity, including their social, cultural, ethnic and religious backgrounds;
2. taking full account of users' needs, whilst recognising that with limited resources it may not always be possible to meet them;
3. providing care and support in ways which are least restrictive to users' liberty and rights. (Department of Health and Welsh Office, 1990).

In addition to the general skills and knowledge discussed elsewhere, post-qualification training should give the ASW a basic knowledge of psychiatry, mental illness, 'normal' and 'abnormal' psychology and emotional disturbances, available treatments, and medication and their effects. It also gives an understanding of how people may react when they are under pressure or feel threatened; patience, calmness and self-assurance in potentially volatile situations and an ability to contain the disturbed feelings of a person experiencing mental distress is essential, for users to feel as safe and confident as possible. As good communication between worker and user is the factor which may determine success or failure in the relationship, an awareness of potential barriers to communication should be present. These barriers may include the effects of treatment or drugs; misunderstandings based on differences in hearing and speech; and the nature of the illness or behavioural disorder (Department of Health and Welsh Office, 1990).

### The appropriate interview

Specific consideration must be given to the process of assessing and interviewing people in mental distress. The Department of Health and Welsh Office (1990: section 2.11) offer a blueprint of good practice which is transferable to all work with adults.

Adequately preparing for the interview by objectively evaluating the reliability of information gathered from a range of sources and considering where and how the interview should take place is essential. The choice of venue should be as comfortable, relaxed and safe as possible. Account must be taken of the user's wishes regarding who should be present at the interview, and potential risks for users, workers and others should be anticipated and evaluated. As far as possible, the interview should involve direct face-to-face contact with the user and adopt a client-centred approach that should involve 'checking out' information in a sensitive and clear way, taking relevant cultural factors into account rather than making assumptions, and utilising interpreters where appropriate.

An awareness of the stresses which may be experienced by those involved with the user, particularly where there are conflicts of interests regarding the safety and protection of family, neighbours or others, is important. A balance must be struck between protecting someone in mental distress from self-harm or from harming others, and enabling them to have maximum control and autonomy over their lives. Although this is difficult for social workers, they need both to understand and to apply their often conflicting roles as carers and agents of social control. That is to say, at times workers may be advocating or protecting users' rights, and at others they may be instrumental in restricting or removing those rights.

In addition to the views of the user, ASWs must take account of those of the nearest relative, and medical and psychiatric opinions (Department of Health and Welsh Office, 1990). Again, where there are different and conflicting perspectives, workers may be placed under extreme pressure regarding other people's or professionals' judgements, and will need to maintain both their objectivity and a good working relationship with those significant others in order to safeguard users' rights and ensure that intervention is guided by reliable information. Any form of intervention or decisions taken must be based on a holistic assessment which takes into account a user's needs in the context of their whole life. Given the discrimination, prejudice and fear operating in society in relation to mental illness, the values of equality, fairness and a commitment to individuals' human rights and worth are essential (Rogers and Pilgrim, 1989), whilst at the same the rights of others not to be put at risk must be considered, as well as guarded.

Arrangements for the care and support of people when discharged from hospital are set out in the *Care Programme Approach* (Department of Health and Welsh Office, 1990), and any support needed will be identified, planned and negotiated with a wide range of agencies.

While the 'Care Programme Approach' (CPA) goes some way to ensure that some patients receive coordinated support form a named 'keyworker' on their discharge, more support is needed in the community for users and those close to them. Inadequate support for those recently discharged from hospital can impact on issues such as their employment, homelessness and readmission, and can contribute to the stress experienced by those to whom users return for their main support in the community (Hatfield and Lefley, 1987). At the same time, the protection of the public from the risk of harm is an essential requirement. This is a serious issue and has been the major criticism of community care since the 1950s. More recently, and following a number of attacks by discharged patients in the community, a serious crisis in mental health services has been identified by a government-appointed Mental Health Task Force (Laurance, 1994). The task force argues that many patients are being discharged without adequate supervision or the provision necessary to meet their housing, social and health needs. This failure increases risk to both the patient and the public.

## Diversion from compulsion and compliance with the law

Where possible, the needs of people in mental distress should be met by care and support in the community rather than by admission to hospital, and the likely long-term effects of compulsory admission on a person's life should be evaluated (Department of Health and Welsh Office, 1990).

Certain factors must be taken into account when an alternative to hospitalisation, compulsory or voluntary, is considered. These must include an understanding of the effect non-admission would have on users and those close to them; ensuring that the need for protection of all those involved is considered; and the range and appropriateness of alternative supports or treatment available should be assessed (Department of Health and Welsh Office, 1990).

Consideration must be given to whether the user would accept medical treatment in hospital voluntarily, or as an out-patient, and there must be an awareness of the dilemmas relating to the extent to which users have real choice. In high-risk situations, if users do not choose voluntary admission, they may be compulsorily admitted. For some people who have voluntarily admitted themselves to hospital, when they attempt to leave before the professionals involved are in agreement, they may be subject to an application compelling them to stay.

Guardianship, though under-used, is arguably the least restrictive order which can be applied for under the Mental Health Act 1983, yet it too is open to criticism as being impossible to implement, given the lengthy process it may involve and the lack of legal powers to ensure that individuals comply with its requirements.

In addition, given that some people experiencing mental distress may come into contact with the criminal justice system, a knowledge of this system and of the theories and research relating to crime and deviance are needed to fully advocate for the user's welfare (see Chapter 6 in this volume).

Community care has created the opportunity for more flexible alternatives to compulsion under the law for people experiencing mental distress. The assessment and care planning process offers a structure within which alternatives to admission or prosecution can be planned and framed more effectively and creatively. The development of budgets has given workers more scope to arrange appropriate resources to meet individuals' needs. If, for instance, a person is likely to need intensive support, it could be arranged for someone with appropriate experience to stay with them in their own home, rather than having to admit them to hospital. Creative planning and implementation of the most appropriate action or services to meet the diverse needs of the individual user is essential.

### Adult/elder abuse

Until recently, the area of adult/elder abuse, and work with affected individuals, was largely neglected. However, interest and concerns have been expressed, and these concerns have been highlighted by coverage in the media and a series of publications (see, for instance, Breckman and Adelman, 1988; Eastman, 1985; Hudson, 1989).

Calls for changes in the law to protect the 'helpless victims' of this abuse, and the use of such value-laden words, may portray and promote the 'dependency culture', and amplify the stereotype of a weak individual unable to make decisions about or be in control of his/her life. In its broadest definition abuse can encompass that of a financial, physical, sexual, psychological or emotional nature, and can be individual or institutionalised. There is no doubt that those experiencing abuse need support, and in some instances protection from the perpetrators. However, as a society and as workers, if social workers ultimately decide to intervene, they need to be clear about why and how they go about achieving that intervention, and on what values they base that decision.

It is important that they have an awareness and understanding of the wider context in which abuse, and elder abuse, can occur and that this is considered in the light of the ageism and discrimination which operates and affects elders, adults and the individuals with whom they are involved.

The stereotypically ageist, Western view of elders regards them as an homogeneous group of people who no longer have, or desire to have, an active or influential role to play in society, and who experience increasing physical and mental decline, most often associated with a belief in their correspondingly decreasing quality of life and worth. This blatantly negative and discriminating view, as with other forms of oppression, creates a climate which contributes to the feelings of powerlessness which elders may experience, promoting the dependency culture which, in turn, is created and reinforced by wider economic and social factors.

Townsend (1981) speaks of the 'structured dependency' of elders, which he argues is a result of older people's experience of forced exclusion from work, and their consequent poverty and institutionalisation, as well as the restricted roles society affords them within their families and in the wider community. Elders and their carers experience and are affected by these negative messages and, given that wherever there is an imbalance of power that power is open to abuse, such a dependency culture may promote an environment in which abuse is likely to occur.

There is no question that carers, and those they care for, can often experience extreme stress and demands which are emotionally and physically exhausting. Hicks (1988) notes that a significant percentage of carers are physically disabled or older people themselves. Similarly, inadequate or inappropriately adapted housing, poverty and isolation of users and carers may all be contributory factors towards an abusive situation or relationship. An awareness of the stresses and frustration carers may experience is important, not to excuse the abuse but, through identifying potential contributory factors or risk indicators, to offer speedy and appropriate support to alleviate or change the situation.

Workers' interventions should always be the least intrusive and most empowering for the user and should be made at an early stage if they are to prevent situations from becoming abusive. A 'solution' approach, which is based on the mechanisms both users and carers positively employ to cope and survive in these situations, builds on individuals' strengths and successes and is more empowering than an approach which concentrates negatively on the apparent difficulties and failings involved.

At some point, where possible, users and carers should be interviewed separately and given the opportunity, in as safe, relaxed and comfortable an environment as possible, to discuss any concerns or fears they may have. However this may not be possible or safe for a range of reasons including carer's and user's distrust of the motivation of the worker, or if they fear that the user may be forced to leave their home. If abuse is occurring, the carer may have obvious concerns regarding the consequences of such an interview for him/her; or users may experience conflicts between their loyalty towards their carer, their dependence upon them for assistance and their fear of possible reprisals should they speak out. Consequently, workers must be aware that their interventions may even *increase the risk* of abuse to users and must act carefully and sensitively. Users and carers may require a range of supports, including access to domiciliary services, respite and day care, carers' centres, financial support, medical treatment, advocates, counselling and legal advice. Users must be given as much information as possible on alternatives and supports available if they are to be enabled to make informed decisions regarding the choices open to them. Where they are unaware of their best interests, or do not know how to mobilise others to act for them, workers must be aware of their responsibilities and act according to appropriate assessments and decisions which incorporate the active participation of users. The point to be made here is that, as Iveson (1990) argues and as has been the main theme of this chapter, empowerment not just protection should be the aim.

## Conclusion

This chapter has attempted to offer an historical and social context of working with adults, the background to community care, the implementation of community care, and the role of social workers within this area of work. User involvement was explored and a consistent theme emerged throughout the chapter: that users need not only be assisted to receive satisfactory services, but also be *empowered* to participate and make choices, as appropriate, with regard to their own lives and, indeed, destiny. As the issues covered in this chapter demonstrate, the knowledge, skills and values of social work as discussed in previous chapters and exemplified in CCETSW (1995) are those most suited to achieve competent work with adults: to working in partnership with users and to enabling them to access the assistance and support they may need.

## References

Barclay P.M. (1982) *Social Workers: Their Role and Tasks*. London: National Institute of Social Work, Bedford Square Press (Barclay Report).

Becker, H.S. (1963) *Outsides: Studies in the Sociology of Deviance*. Chicago: Free Press.

Breckman, R. and Adelman, R. (1988) *Strategies for Helping Victims of Elder Mistreatment*. London: Sage.

Brown, R. (1987) *The Approved Social Workers Guide to the Mental Health Act 1983*. London: Community Care/Reed Business Publishing.

CCETSW (1991) *DipSW: Rules and Requirements for the Diploma in Social Work* (Paper 30), 2nd edn. London: Central Council for Education and Training in Social Work.

CCETSW (1995) *DipSW: Rules and Requirements for the Diploma in Social Work* (Paper 30), revised edn. London: Central Council for Education and Training in Social Work.

Centre for Policy on Ageing (1990) *Community Life: A Code of Practice for Community Care*. London: CPA.

Davies, A. (1982) *Women, Race and Class*. London: The Women's Press.

Department of Health (1989) *Caring for People: Community Care in the Next Decade and Beyond*. London: HMSO.

Department of Health (1991a) *Care Management and Assessment: Manager's Guide*. London: HMSO.

Department of Health (1991b) *Care Management and Assessment: Practitioner's Guide*. London: HMSO.

Department of Health and Social Security (1968) *Report of the Committee on Local Authority and Allied Social Services* (Seebohm Report). London: HMSO.

Department of Health and Welsh Office (1990) *Code of Practice – Mental Health Act 1983*. London: HMSO.

Donlan, P. (1993) 'Empowerment and quality in community care', in V. Williamson (ed.), *Users First*. Brighton: University of Brighton Press.

Downes, D. and Rock, P. (1988) *Understanding Deviance: A Guide to the Sociology of Crime and Rule Breaking*, 2nd edn. Oxford: Oxford University Press.

Eastman, M. (1985) *Old Age Abuse*. London: Age Concern.

Egan, G. (1986) *The Skilled Helper: A Systematic Approach to Effective Helping*, 3rd edn. Pacific Grove, CA: Brooks/Cole.

Erikson, E. (1982) *The Life Cycle Completed*. New York: Norton.

Fanon, F. (1967) *The Wretched Earth*. Harmondsworth: Penguin.

Finch, J. and Groves, D. (1980) 'Community care and the family: a case for equal opportunities?', *Journal of Social Policy*, 9(4): 486–511.

Finch, J. and Groves, D. (eds) (1983) *A Labour of Love: Women, Work and Caring*. London: Routledge.

Fishwick, C. (1992) *Community Care and Control: a Guide to the Legislation*. Birmingham: PEPAR.

George, M. and Lineham, T. (1994) 'Two nations', *Community Care*, 18–24 August: 14–15.

Goffman, E. (1961) *Asylums: Essays on the Social Situation of Mental Patients and Other Inmates*. New York: Doubleday.

Griffiths, R. (1988) *Community Care: Agenda for Action*. London: HMSO.

Haslett, C. (1991) 'The Children Act 1989 and community care: comparisons and contrasts', *Policy and Politics*, 19(4): 283–91.

Hatfield, A.B. and Lefley, H.P. (eds) (1987) *Families of the Mentally Ill – Coping and Adaptation*. London: Cassell Educational.

Hicks, C. (1988) *Who Care: Looking after People at Home*. London: Virago.

Hudson, M. (1989) 'Analyses of the concepts of elder mistreatment: abuse and neglect', *Journal of Elder Abuse and Neglect*, 1: 5–26.

Iveson, C. (1990) *Whose Life? Community Care of Older People and their Families*. London: Brief Therapy Press.

Laing, R.D. (1967) *The Politics of Experience*. Harmondsworth: Penguin.

Laurance, J. (1994) 'Mental care crisis "puts public and patients at risk"', *Times*, 28 September.

Lishman, J. (ed. (1991) *Handbook of Theory for Practice Teachers in Social Work*. London: Jessica Kingsley.

May, T. and Vass, A.A. (eds) (1996) *Working with Offenders: Issues, Contexts and Outcomes*. London: Sage.

Morris, J. (1991) *Pride against Prejudice: Transforming Attitudes to Disability*. London: The Women's Press.

Morris, J. (1993) *Community Care or Independent Living?* York: Joseph Rowntree Foundation.

Ogden, J. (1994) 'DSS "inflated" cost of disability bill', *Care Weekly*, 328: 6.

Oliver, M (ed.) (1993) *Social Work with Disabled People*. Basingstoke: Macmillan.

Rogers, A. and Pilgrim, D. (1989) 'Mental health and citizenship', *Critical Social Policy*, 9(2): 44–55.

Rowlings, C. (1981) *Social Work with Ageing People*. London: Allen & Unwin.

Smale, G., Tuson, G., Biehal, N. and Marsh, P. (1993) *Empowerment, Assessment, Care Management and the Skilled Worker*. London: National Institute of Social Work/HMSO.

Smith, D. (1995) *Criminology for Social Work*. London: Macmillan.

Stevenson, O. and Parsloe, P. (1993) *Community Care and Empowerment*. York: Joseph Rowntree Foundation.

Tinker, A. (1984) *The Elderly in Modern Society*, London: Longman.

Townsend, P. (1981) 'The structured dependency of the elderly: creation of social policy in the twentieth century', *Ageing and Social Policy*, 1(1): 5–28.

Vass, A.A. (1990) *Alternatives to Prison: Punishment, Custody and the Community*. London: Sage.

Vass, A.A. and Taylor, J. (1995) 'Re-inventing practice: practitioners' perceptions of change following the National Health Service and Community Care Act 1990', unpublished paper, London: School of Social Work and Health Sciences, Middlesex University.

Wertheimer, A. (1993) 'User participation in community care: the challenge for services', in V. Williamson (ed.), *Users First: The Real Challenge for Community Care*. Brighton: University of Brighton Press.

# 6

# Crime, Probation and Social Work with Offenders

This chapter covers the core knowledge, values and skills required in working with offenders. In the limited space available it is not possible to cover issues in much detail and the reader is advised to consult other relevant texts (see for instance CCETSW, 1995:23–36; Geary, 1994; Home Office et al., 1995; Hungerford-Welch, 1994; Jones et al., 1992; May and Vass, 1996; Raynor et al., 1994; Sprack, 1992; Ward and Ward, 1993; Williams, 1994; Wasik, 1993; Wasik and Taylor, 1991).

The major duties and tasks of those working with offenders in a formal and regular capacity as well as the current sentencing options for the supervision and punishment of offenders in the community are set out in the Probation Rules (1984) and by several Acts of Parliament. Probation was first recognised in statute in 1907. The Powers of Criminal Courts Act 1973 consolidated previous enactments on probation orders and introduced the community service order. The Criminal Justice Act 1991 further extended the range of community penalties, made the probation order for the first time a sentence of the court (rather than an alternative to a sentence) and set them all within a common framework.

Those who work with offenders are faced with considerable challenge and constant change. For example, services are responding to important and significant initiatives, such as changes in training (Nellis, 1996), emphasis on competences (Boswell, 1996), dramatic changes in criminal justice (Home Office, 1995a; Smith, 1996; Vass, 1996), tackling discrimination (Denney, 1996), developing partnerships with other agencies (Broad, 1996; Gilling, 1996) and questions about service provision and its effectiveness (Mair et al., 1994; Lloyd et al., 1994; Raynor, 1996).

In the above social context of fast-changing social relationships and requirements guiding the work of social workers and probation officers in dealing with offenders, 'Competition for scarce resources means that day-to-day performance is increasingly under scrutiny and services must now demonstrate value for money in terms that the public can understand' (Probation Training Unit, 1994:vii). Within that framework of social, legal, economic, political and organisational change, the operation and performance of probation and social services personnel (in the case of supervision of juveniles by local authorities) are monitored and subject to inspection by HM Inspectorate of Probation (HM Inspectorate of Probation, 1993, 1994) and the Social Services Inspectorate respectively. Required standards of practice to which all forms of formal intervention and supervision are expected to comply are set by the government in the form of 'national standards'. *National Standards for the Supervision of Offenders in the Community* was first published in 1992 (Home Office et al., 1992) and extensively revised in 1995 (Home Office et al., 1995). At the same time, in order to ensure that those who work with offenders are to improve their performance in the above challenging climate, an emphasis has been placed, rightly or wrongly (see May and Vass 1996 for a critical account), on the development and enhancement of 'competences' (CCETSW, 1995:23–36; Probation Training Unit, 1994).

Crudely, a simple definition of 'competence' is 'the ability to perform work activities to the expected standard' (Probation Training Unit, 1994:1). This means that 'Increasingly, judgements of individual capability are being based on the ability to meet the measurable requirements of a job rather than on the more general criteria of experience, qualifications or background' (Probation Training Unit, 1994:1). The benefits which are assumed to accrue from defining standards and conforming to them are both individual and organisational. At the individual level, competences make important 'contributions to recognising . . . effectiveness and pride in [one's] work. . . . Expertise can be more readily transferred and movement between jobs and services facilitated' (Probation Training Unit, 1994:2). At the organisational level, 'Management systems based on competences lead to fairer, more effective organisations with greater staff satisfaction. The notion of competence brings a new approach to supporting individual staff members, and helping them develop their potential' (Probation Training Unit, 1994:2).

Although the above claims are somewhat flawed (see Boswell, 1996; Nellis, 1996) for they present competences as something which can be learned by anyone on the spot by following through guidelines which are formulated in the form of a shopping list of 'dos and don'ts' (a caricature, and dangerous at that, of what standards, quality and performance stand for), the essence of being competent ought to be about defining and combining knowledge, values and skills which can be applied and transferred if need be from one context to another, and from one job to another.

In that sense, competence is the ability to perform in diverse contexts and with offenders from diverse backgrounds, sentences, dispositions and needs. It is the ability to understand, assess and make choices (hence reach decisions) by utilising and combining knowledge, values, skills and experience.

## The purpose of the probation service

The probation service serves the courts and the public by supervising offenders in the community; helping offenders to lead law-abiding lives that minimise risk to the public; and safeguarding the welfare of children in family proceedings.

Those who work with offenders are expected to undertake a number of major tasks and meet responsibilities which are basically to provide the courts with information and advice, as appropriate, on offenders to assist in sentencing decisions; to implement community penalties passed by courts; to design, provide and promote effective programmes for the supervision of offenders in the community; to assist prisoners before and after release, to lead law-abiding lives; to help communities prevent, cope with and reduce crime and its effects on victims; to reconcile the needs of offenders and communities, recognising the obligations of both and the need to manage risk safely; to provide information to the courts on the best interests of children in family disputes; to work in partnership with other bodies and services in using the most appropriate and constructive methods of dealing with offenders and defendants.

The role of those who work with offenders is to aim at controlling and reducing crime. In so doing, they are required to deliver the best possible quality of service by recognising that the individuals with whom they work have rights and responsibilities and that differences among those individuals are acknowledged in a positive manner. Workers should establish effective working relationships with service users, other agencies and the community at large, and ensure that all relevant procedures and statutory requirements are followed and complied with. All service users should expect to be treated fairly, openly and with respect, and information about them should be treated in a confidential manner and in accordance with the law and relevant codes of practice. Finally, those working with offenders are publicly accountable for their actions and need to maintain high standards of service if they are to earn the confidence of the public, courts and individual service users (CCETSW, 1995; Probation Training Unit, 1994).

## Values

It is evident from the above that if the aims of meeting the challenges and complexities of working with offenders, often in conditions of considerable tension, conflict and ambiguity (for instance, reconciling the needs of offenders and those of the community), a set of values need to be adhered to and used as a guiding force in dealing with service users. Within the above responsibilities and expectations there are clear indications and references to what those values are and should be.

In the main, working with offenders may not be so different from generally dealing with individuals whose needs or problems fall outside criminal law. That is to say, probation officers and others who work with offenders share the main social work values of assisting 'people to have control of and improve the quality of their lives and are committed to reducing and preventing hardship and disadvantage for children, adults, families and groups' (CCETSW, 1995:4). They deal, as do social workers in general, with individuals and social settings characterised by diversity. 'This diversity is reflected through religion, ethnicity, culture, language, social status, family structure and life style' (CCETSW, 1995:4). Given that their actions have serious implications on users and the community, probation officers, like social workers, must treat people with respect, be trustworthy and efficient. As the chapter on skills has argued, they must also be 'self-aware and critically reflective' (see also CCETSW, 1995:4). Their practice, therefore, must be 'founded on, informed and capable of being judged against a clear value base' (CCETSW, 1995:4).

CCETSW (1995:4) summarises this value base thus:

- Workers identify and question their own values and prejudices and the implications of these for practice.
- They respect and value uniqueness and diversity, and recognise and build on strengths.
- They promote people's rights to choice, privacy, confidentiality and protection, while recognising and addressing the complexities of competing rights and demands.
- They assist people to increase control of and improve the quality of their lives, while recognising that control of behaviour will be required at times in order to protect children and adults from harm.
- They identify, analyse and take action to counter discrimination, racism, disadvantage, inequality and injustice, using strategies appropriate to role and context.
- They practise in a manner that does not stigmatise or disadvantage individuals, groups or communities.

Converting the above general values into more specific probation and offender-oriented work, they can be summarised thus:

- Workers challenge attitudes and behaviour which result in crime and cause distress, or harm to victims and others.
- They reconcile the needs of offenders and communities, recognising the obligations of both and the need to manage risk safely.
- They treat all service users fairly, openly and with respect, and promote and maintain anti-discriminatory practice.
- They work at all times to bring out the best in people.
- They recognise that the individuals with whom they work have rights and responsibilities.
- They are publicly accountable.

When those values are considered together, that is to say the general values together with the specific ones, the emphasis is on five notions of personal and social responsibility: *respect for persons, care for persons, hope for the future* (see Bottoms and Stelman, 1988: ch. 3), *community cohesion* and *social justice* (Bottoms, 1989). Respecting the person means that the offender's 'capacity as a free person to make choices, including sometimes choices that the probation officer might not like' (Bottoms, 1989:44) is recognised. Recognising the person's choices and caring for that individual at the same time requires that the offender is considered a whole person and not just someone who has committed an offence. Building on that, the value of hope becomes important for it 'sees possibilities even in the most unlikely individuals and social situations' (Bottoms, 1989:44). Community cohesion arises because 'it is desirable that the various elements in our society should relate to one another with reasonable harmony' and social justice is closely related to that, 'since it is difficult to espouse the concept of "community cohesion" in a grossly unjust society' (Bottoms, 1989:44).

In addition to these core values, it is necessary to add the value of *confronting crime* – challenging offenders to accept responsibility for their actions – and to become aware of the impact of crime on victims. In short, the above values do not, and should not, exclude the necessary administration and application of controls and censorship if they are required.

As said earlier, there may be a distinct impression that there are serious contradictions between caring, say, for offenders and at the same time aiming at controlling them; or caring for the offender and at the same time caring for the community. However, we believe this dichotomy has been exaggerated in the field of probation and any other social setting involving the supervision of offenders in the community. As has been argued elsewhere, who says care says control (Vass, 1984; see also Harris, 1980, 1988). It is not inherently contradictory to control and care for someone. This is evident in all 'normal' social relationships where an element of care versus control, love and hate, usually coexist and indeed are necessary parts of any meaningful social encounter. There is no reason to believe that this duality between what are seen to be opposing values cannot be reconciled to engender a fair, efficient and just service. As Bottoms (1989:44) puts it:

> there is nothing inherently contradictory in the idea of a social work agency exercising certain control functions. Indeed, social work in other contexts [other than offenders], such as child care, does quite overtly undertake various controlling actions. The debate on this particular subject seems to me to have become unhelpfully polarised, and not really assisted by the rhetoric either of the pro-social work/anti-control lobby or the pro-control/anti-social work lobby. The real issue, as it seems to me, is whether any particular suggested sanction, or any proposed method of enforcement, is incompatible with any of the . . . core social work values.

Furthermore, without negotiating and reconciling the interests of individuals generally, the maintenance and cohesion of the community, and the interests of offenders themselves it is not possible to exercise action which is meaningful to all concerned. If it is not meaningful but demeaning, one cannot refer to respect for individuals, fairness and justice and so on. A particularly revealing paragraph which explains the necessity to exercise social work values as specified earlier occurs in a lecture by the late Archbishop Temple (cited in Bottoms, 1989:44–5) who said:

> The community has three interests to consider: first, the maintenance of its own life and order, upon which the welfare of all its members depends; secondly, the interest of the individual members generally; and thirdly, the interest of the offending member himself. I believe that this is the true, indeed the necessary, order of priority. But wrong is done if any of the three is neglected. In particular it is to be noticed that though the interest of the offender comes last, yet if this be neglected, the action taken loses its quality of punishment and deteriorates into vengence, for the offender is then no longer treated as within the society that takes penal action, but over against it, and therefore outside it.

The 'key point', as Bottoms (1989:45) suggests, is 'that the defendant "never is only criminal and nothing else", and that any human society demeans itself if it treats him as if he were nothing else'. This is why it is relevant to value the belief that all people have something 'better' or 'more' to offer and why one should be working at all times to bring out the best in people.

The reference to anti-discriminatory practice is of particular relevance here. One cannot afford respect to others or treat them fairly and in a just manner or help them to bring out the best in themselves if they are being discriminated against. In keeping with the duty not to discriminate referred to in section 95 of the Criminal Justice Act 1991, the work of probation services, social services departments and all those with whom they work in partnership, should be free of discrimination on the ground of race, gender, age, disability, language ability, literacy, religion, sexual orientation or any other improper ground. Where language difficulties impair effective communication with an offender an accredited interpreter should be used. In Wales, an offender should have the right to use Welsh, if necessary through an interpreter (Home Office et al., 1995:5–6). It must be noted, however, that although section 95 of the Criminal Justice Act 1991 requires the Secretary of State to publish information for the purposes of 'facilitating the avoidance of discrimination on the grounds of race or sex or any other improper ground', this does not constitute a statutory duty (Ward and Ward, 1993:4). As Ward and Ward (1993:4) add:

> it cannot therefore be relied upon directly to challenge the actions or decisions of those within the criminal justice system. However, it does constitute a statutory recognition of this important principle. Practitioners should ensure that assessments of seriousness levels avoid any disparity of treatment or stereotypical judgements. This will also be important in assessing the suitability of a particular community order, and which requirements (if any) are imposed.

Exercising anti-discriminatory practice cannot rely just on statements of intent, guidelines and procedures. It depends, to a greater extent, on how individual workers choose to work with service users. It is worth reminding the reader of the basic values which are essential in ensuring a determined and consistent approach to combating overt and covert forms of discrimination:

- Workers must know themselves, by identifying and questioning their own values and prejudices and the implications of these for practice.
- They need to accept uniqueness and diversity and recognise and build on strengths.
- They need to accept and respect individual rights and circumstances and understand how these affect the delivery of services to offenders and communities.
- They must learn to counter discrimination, racism, poverty, disadvantage and injustice in ways appropriate to the situation and their role.
- They must eliminate discrimination and disadvantage in all aspects of their work.

• They must remain publicly accountable and demonstrate anti-discriminatory practice through the quality assurance process.


## Knowledge

Chapter 1 in this volume described at some length the various areas of knowledge that social workers and probation officers need to cover in order to be competent in their practice – for example the historical context of social work, social science perspectives and their application to practice, power relationships, components of effective communication with children, young people, adults, groups and communities, theories and models of social work, concepts of empowerment, research and its implications for practice, statutory duties and assessment of need (see also, CCETSW, 1995). The knowledge base needed for working with offenders shares the same general knowledge required and expected of social workers. However, as an area of practice, working with offenders has, in addition, its own specific body of knowledge which provides insights and understanding of offending, organisational matters including the function of and interconnections of constituent parts of the criminal justice system, sentencing and range of penal sanctions, roles, tasks and requirements, and effectiveness of intervention amongst others. A detailed and critical discussion of these issues, and others, and how they relate to effective practice has been covered elsewhere (see May and Vass, 1996). In this section we cover particular aspects, albeit in brief, of this knowledge base which is essential to everyone working for the probation service, social services departments, the voluntary or independent sectors and whose main responsibilities include the supervision of offenders or who may have some other direct or indirect involvement in criminal justice. It is often wrongly assumed that only probation officers require this knowledge base, as social workers have little to do with criminal justice. This is a very unfortunate and unhelpful myth which has led to both poor knowledge (as information about crime and criminal justice is deemed to be irrelevant) and poor practices. For example, every competent social worker must be in a position to understand courts and how they work, write reports for them (e.g. pre-sentence reports) and know what sentencing options are available at the time to make an informed judgement. Indeed, national standards for the supervision of offenders place responsibilities not only on the probation service but also on every social services department in the country (Home Office et al., 1995).

*Criminology, crime and deviance*

This is a vast field which covers many controversial issues, including the historical context, definitions and the criminal process, statistics and implications for policy, public conceptions and misconceptions about crime, victims and victimisation, theories (from biological and psychological to social), feminist criminology, crime, fear of crime, crime prevention and the community (including inter-agency work), crime and mental health, lifestyle, accommodation and employment, race and crime. There are many texts which cover the general topic or specific aspects of this area and it is expected that individuals working with offenders must have a basic knowledge and understanding of relevant issues (see, for instance, Downes and Rock, 1988; Smith, 1995; Williams, 1994). We agree with Smith (1995:1) when he writes:

> much of this work [criminology] can and should be understood in a way which makes it usable as practical knowledge, sometimes directly, as when empirical work is used to inform changes in practice; sometimes indirectly, as part of a broader process of 'enlightenment' . . . which leads to changes in professional aims, values and culture. . . . Criminology is essentially an applied discipline, a helping science, which positively ought to engage with the problems which confront practitioners in the criminal justice 'system' (if it can be called that), and with the problems of crime and its effects, which thousands of lay people experience every day – as offenders, as victims or as citizens concerned about the impact of crime on themselves, their families or their neighbourhoods, or society as a whole.

It is important to emphasise that studying criminology and theories of crime does not in itself offer ready-made solutions to crime. There are reasons for this. Each theory and model of crime (and hence society) offers a version of what *might* be 'reality' but 'proof' remains, for all of them, a very elusive and unaccomplished task. There are too many complex and intertwined (known and unknown) environmental, political, psychological, social and other variables at play for criminology to come up with clear and distinct answers to questions about crime and its prevention. As such, much of the knowledge in this area is subjective in that proof is based on interpretative knowledge accrued by surveys, observation, armchair theorisation, and reviews or reassessment of available information and on the perspectives of the interpreters. For example, the relationship between unemployment and crime may appear to be incontestable in the context of rising unemployment and crime in the 1980s and 1990s (see Dickinson, 1993; Farrington et al., 1986; Field, 1990). But the debate whether unemployment causes crime (or whether some other variable is involved which contributes to higher rates of crimes in specific settings and by specific social or age groups) or whether crime itself leads to higher levels of unemployment (by excluding individuals from competing in the market economy) continues unabated. As Williams (1994:285) writes, 'There is now widespread, though not total, acceptance that there is a strong relationship between criminality and economic or income inequality; that there is probably a relationship between crime and unemployment; and that this relationship is strongest in the case of young males', but there are conflicting accounts and interpretations of that relationship and how it affects a society (for a review of various claims see Williams, 1994:282–5). The common counter-argument is that poverty, economic or income inequality and unemployment cannot be regarded as causes of crime as there are many people who experience deprivation (are materially poor and without regular or any employment) but do not appear to commit crimes. The counter-argument, in its simplest form, suggests, therefore, that crime does not relate to the absolute levels of poverty or wealth in a given society. On the other hand, though, an equally rational and persuasive argument is that in a fairer and more egalitarian society some forms of crime (property offences) could be reduced.

Part of the problem in discussing crime and its prevention is that people often take the concept of crime for granted without realising that it is both difficult to define in any concrete way and extremely hard to measure. Something which is normally forgotten is that we refer to crime in the singular when in fact we should refer to 'crimes'. Our perceptions and understanding are clouded by a failure to distinguish between different types and acts of crime in discussions, debates and policies. Secondly, references to crime are normally made as if everyone knows what constitutes crime and that common sense tells us what is criminal and non-criminal. That is far from the truth. It may sound far-fetched for some but there is no definition of crime which can be put to universal application. Crime and its definitions cannot be separated from the societal context, the legal system, and normative evaluations of behaviour and actions. The definition of acts as criminal or deviant depends largely on two sets of related norms: the legal and the moral codes prevailing at the time (for such codes change with time) in any society. In moral terms many acts can be unacceptable and deviant but may not be criminal. They can only be criminal if an act of human behaviour is barred by criminal law. If that act is committed and breaks a legal rule, it is deemed to be an offence. An offence, though, may not be criminal unless the law says so. But laws (including criminal law) which have universal application and legitimacy in a society like

England and Wales are enacted by the apparatus of the state. Inevitably, it is politicians given ministerial power (following personal choice or advice from competing interests), Parliament, and interpretations of the law by judges which define and constitute acts as criminal. Williams (1994:11) summarises these ambiguities about crime and the role of the state very succinctly:

> it is essential that one never forgets that no matter how immoral, reprehensible, damaging or dangerous an act is, it is not a crime unless it is made such by the authorities of the State – the legislature and, at least through interpretation, the judges.

Thirdly, there is a criminal process of proving guilt which has to be completed before even an act which violates a criminal code of conduct can be deemed to be criminal. That is to say, breaking the law may be seen to be criminal but it is not officially designated as such until formal conviction. It is the *act* which is in question. Conviction implies that in court it was found that the person involved had *acted* against the law (i.e. the *actus reus* of the crime). Persons may commit acts which violate the law but, in defence, they may prove that they had acted lawfully. Crime, therefore, and the process of defining acts as criminal, involves procedural rules, 'scripts', 'roles' and 'parts' to follow and 'play' by many individuals in the system before the legality or illegality of an act is established. Playing 'crime games', as in playing 'war games', involves a measure of ceremony, ritualism and theatrical presentation before any outcomes are announced. Within that social context of becoming criminal, the procedural script is normally followed rather rigidly but the 'story' and how that story or drama unfolds and is played out by participants remains by and large unpredictable until the defendant is found guilty or not guilty. Furthermore, in the context of deliberations, and in most court cases, the intentions of the individual in committing the act, whether he or she intended to commit the crime (i.e. *mens rea*), are considered. For example, in a recent case an Algerian asylum-seeker who attacked a doctor after being told to stop smoking at a London underground station was sentenced to 21 months' imprisonment. After sentencing him, the judge in the case said he would not make a recommendation for deportation and explained this decision thus:

> Courts have a duty to try to protect innocent members of the public going about their normal business on the Underground and unless courts take a very firm view of wholly unprovoked violence of this kind then they are failing in their duty. . . . This offence, though extremely serious, was not pre-planned but something that flared up at that moment and I

don't think this is a case where I should make a recommendation for deportation. (quoted in *Independent*, 1995)

As can be observed, as the act, 'though extremely serious' and 'unprovoked', was not 'pre-planned' (hence, unpremeditated), the more serious consequence for the offender – deportation – was withheld. However, this idea of not planning to commit a crime and not recognising its consequences does not always lead to such leniency or a consistent (non-discriminatory) interpretation of intent. Occasionally it can lead to injustices against women who suffer a history of mental and physical abuse at the hands of their male spouses or acquaintances. After years of experiencing such abuse, some women are led to despair and commit violent crimes against their male partners which sometimes result in their death or serious injury. In such cases, the issue of *mens rea* can work against women if courts take the view that the crime *was* the result of a history of mental and physical abuse. As there was a history to the crime, unlike the spontaneous combustion which led to the violent crime in the earlier example, the implication can be that the commission of the act was not the result of a reaction which 'flared up at that moment' but a crime which was premeditated: that the defendant had planned the method and the timing (whilst, say, the man was incapacitated – drunk or asleep – and thus defenceless). Indeed, one of the most common defences against the *mens rea* of an offence, a plea of diminished responsibility or insanity, may not appear convincing in the face of that history of events.

Interpretation of premeditation and intended consequences, therefore, can establish or limit guilt and as such can have an effect on the outcome – how the crime is defined, categorised or punished.

Fourthly, what crime is, is what statistics tell us it is. As storytellers, they do not tell all. They only report offences known to the police and the courts, and sentences passed. It is estimated that only a fraction of acts which breach the law are ever in the public view, so there is much crime which remains hidden: crimes are committed by many more people than statistics would have us believe. Everyone is capable of some form of offence but the difference is whether one is caught or not. Only those who are caught or prosecuted enter the official data which provide a profile of type and incidence of crimes. In that sense, the role of the police, social workers, probation officers and others in defining and socially constructing statistics (by the choices they make and the discretion they exercise in taking action against offenders) is significant. As has been argued elsewhere (see Vass, 1996 for a critical discussion) one of the reasons why offenders given community penalties (e.g.

straight probation orders and community service: see Lloyd et al., 1994) show a slightly lower reconviction rate in comparison to people who are released following imprisonment is that probation officers, like other law enforcers, can influence outcomes by the decisions they take (e.g. to prosecute or not to prosecute defaulters). Similarly, a considerable amount of research in the 1960s, particularly in the USA, about police decisions in apprehending suspects clearly demonstrated that many factors, other than demeanour (e.g. the gender, race, self-presentation, verbal and non-verbal cues and perceived social class of the suspect), play a part in the decision to prosecute or not to prosecute. Recent research postulates that black offenders (Afro-Caribbeans) are proportionately more likely than whites or Asians to be arrested and are more likely to be charged after arrest for offences which run a high risk of imprisonment (Jefferson and Walker, 1992; Walker, 1988, 1989).

Closely connected with the social construction of statistics is the distinction one should draw between *actual* crime and *fear* of crime. Statistics and the way in which those 'facts' are presented or misrepresented by the media can largely colour popular conceptions of crime and the fear of crime. In turn, this fear of crime, and of falling victim to some serious if not violent act, creates a state of siege and leads many groups of people, particularly women and older people, to change their lifestyle in order to protect themselves from harm (Hough and Mayhew, 1985). In terms of statistics, this fear may have very little relation to the actual occurrence of crime and the risk of victimisation. It is young people who consistently appear to be the most vulnerable group, that is, who are more likely to be victimised, and yet they are the ones who, according to crime surveys, express the least fear. This exaggerated (for some social groups) or underestimated (by younger people) fear of falling victim to crime adds to the confusion and somewhat amplifies the complexities of understanding and coping with crime. This is not a new phenomenon for historically it has been demonstrated that crime, definitions of criminal acts, and fear of crime have always been part and parcel of the social structure (Pearson, 1983).

However, it is fundamentally inaccurate and indeed morally wrong to impute meaning to the fact that just because people have unrealistic fears of crime they are, in some way, irrational. For it should be appreciated, as W.I. Thomas (an influential figure in the emergence of symbolic interactionism in its original and unsystematised form) once put it, 'if [people] define situations as real, they are real in their consequences'. What this means is that it does not really matter very much if one is *actually* at risk. If she or he *believes* so, that is a social fact and the effects of that fact are real: not imaginary or irrational. Furthermore, remembering what was said earlier about hidden crime which never comes to the notice of the public or the authorities *other than the private worlds and experiences of victims*, that fear may be a realistic, rational response to an *actual* experience which was not reported. In fact, various authors have raised doubts about claims that fear of crime by some social groups, especially women and members of minority ethnic groups, is an exaggerated affair (see readings in Maguire and Pointing, 1988; Mawby and Walklate, 1994). Work carried out by the Centre for Criminology at Middlesex University (Jones et al., 1986) and other criminologists (Dobash and Dobash, 1980; Stanko, 1987, 1988; Russell, 1982) found that more crimes were committed against women than were normally reported, and that many women knew of acquaintances who had been sexually attacked but had not reported that to the authorities. These findings may imply that, for some groups, fear of crime may be a very realistic assessment of and response to a real risk. These same social groups, including older people and minority ethnic groups, may experience more crime or acts of deviance against them than is commonly accepted or understood, but are effectively suffering in private and in silence.

*Theories of crime and deviance*
Asking the question 'what causes crime' or 'why do people commit crimes' and expecting an absolute or conclusive answer is like searching for the pot of gold at the end of a rainbow. Simply, there is no definite and agreed explanation why people, some more than others, commit criminal offences. There are varied explanations including economic, physical and genetic, biochemical, psychological, sociological and feminist critiques (for a useful discussion of most of these, their contributions, weaknesses and relevance to policy, see Smith, 1995; Williams, 1994). Here we will give brief illustrations of the diversity of approach.

*Economic* explanations question assumptions that offenders are sick, abnormal, deviant, or deprived. Rather, they regard offenders as rational and calculating and, as in normal economic circumstances, trying to maximise their choices and preferences subject to given constraints (which in this instance are taken to be legal codes and fear of punishment). One view is that all individuals have insatiable desires which cannot be accommodated or attained because of limited resources, particularly income. Preferences and tastes differ between individuals, who have different genetic characteristics and are subject to different socioeconomic opportunities. Crudely, individuals calculate their chances of achieving their aspirations through legitimate income; the amount of income offered by these legitimate opportunities; the extra opportunities offered via illicit means; the probability of being apprehended and charged for the illegal dealings; and finally, if caught and punished, what punishment to expect. It is as though a balance sheet is drawn up made up of the assets/benefits (of maximising choice through crime) and costs/liabilities (if found out). It is in this sense that the offender is seen as a normal, calculating individual who conducts a cost/benefit analysis of engaging in crime.

The inevitable conclusion reached, by such an approach, about how to discourage the use of illicit methods of maximising social and economic 'profit' is to increase the chances of the offender being caught, in the first place, and, in the second place, to ensure that she or he will receive severe punishment (e.g. making prisons harsher and more unpleasant).

There is no denying the fact that such an explanation of crime is seductively attractive as it explains something that common sense associates with: greed. Many people are 'greedy' and much of the problem in contemporary society is placed squarely and directly on their appetite for maximising their income and worldly goods. Crime is a means to achieve that goal. The approach is also attractive because it draws little distinction between offenders and others. They are not propelled into situations against their will. They choose to act illicitly and attach meaning to their actions.

However, there are many problems with this sort of explanation. For example, it is relevant to some property offences (including theft from the person) but it is difficult to see how it can explain crimes which are committed for reasons other than economic benefit (e.g. men's crimes against women or 'crimes of passion'). It is also questionable that, even in crimes where economic benefit is considered, people committing those acts are so systematic and calculating and preoccupied with economic budgeting. Much of crime can in fact be opportunistic – relevant to specific moments, settings and circumstances. More seriously, it appears to rely on statistics which normally show an over-representation of individuals from the less affluent sections of society. As said earlier, as opportunities are unequal, some people try to increase their economic chances by illicit techniques, which makes it look as though crime is the prerogative of certain groups in society. As an explanation, it falls short of offering a realistic understanding about 'white-collar crime' such as misrepresentation in financial statements of corporations, manipulation of the Stock Exchange, commercial bribery, bribery of public officials and politicians, embezzlement and misapplication of funds and tax frauds (Sutherland and Cressey, 1966). Many of these activities remain invisible and therefore hidden from statistics. Where they become visible, a large proportion of those who commit such crimes are not convicted in criminal courts. Although one can suggest that the same principle of greed and maximisation of benefits is the guiding force behind such crimes, such individuals have the means and capacity to evade recognition and punishment. When they are recognised, punishment normally falls short of expectation and is disproportionate to the social cost and damage done by their activity.

*Biological/psychological* explanations (see Smith, 1995: ch. 3; Williams, 1994:111–263) emphasise, in the main, the characteristics of the individuals who commit crimes. Such explanations tend to look at their biological make-up, attitudes, emotions, motivations and adaptations or adjustments to the environment, psychosexual development and a host of other intrinsic characteristics.

In biological terms, it is believed that genes play a part in explaining criminality. As people are individually genetically unique (except identical twins) this explains why some commit crimes and others do not though they may experience similar social and sometimes physical environments. In contrast to early biological theories which relied exclusively on genetic factors in explaining crime, contemporary works are more sophisticated and involve the study of both genetics and social influences (Ellis and Hoffman, 1990). In addition, since intrinsic characteristics can be located, it follows that the availability of 'experts' to administer 'treatment' becomes relevant. Williams (1994:111) writes:

> most modern researchers do not view the part played by biology in any explanation of criminality as indicating an illness or a dysfunction; rather it suggests the possibility of a slightly different configuration of normal genes giving rise to a temperament which is more receptive to antisocial types of behaviour. Furthermore many do not view such differences as immutable, recognising instead that biological and genetic differences can be altered.

One particular example, which blends biology, personality and environment, is worth referring to as an illustration. The framework of psychoanalysis has received canonical status and differential interpretations, resulting in the development of diverse psycho-analytic accounts of criminality. Psychoanalytic theory has had a useful but also perverse effect on social work (Pearson et al., 1988; Smith, 1995). Psychoanalytic criminology is already nearly a century old and remains a strong influence on theories of crime.

Psychoanalytic criminology starts out with the crucial assumption that all human behaviour is motivated and thus goal-oriented or teleological in character (Feldman, 1964). Since human behaviour is motivated and goal-oriented, it follows, it is argued, that human behaviour is functional in that it fulfils a desire or need. However, to understand the motives or functions of an act one must not just observe the end product, that is the outcome of the behaviour (overt action), but must understand subjective meanings and the significance which the actors attach to themselves. The principle of subjective understanding (which is dealt with in more detail later in this chapter) is an established tenet in sociological theory and runs in the tradition of Max Weber's *Verstehen*, that is to say the search for meaning. It is an approach which analyses social situations according to how people orient their actions toward one another and which influences their meanings, intentions and behaviour resulting from this action orientation. Psychoanalytic subjective understanding goes a step further and becomes more complex. Psychoanalysis ascertains that the concept of subjective meaning which actors attach to their actions may be unconscious: the actors themselves may be unaware of the functions they impute to their own actions. In essence, an act can have both overt and latent functions. For example, an act of stealing may appear to offer rewards to the thief by the acquisition of the goods so desired but psychoanalytic theory may explain the function at the unconscious level, which may have a deeper meaning and significance. It may, for instance, indicate that the individual committing theft is trying to attract attention to herself or himself, to be apprehended and penalised for some other 'wrong'. Through this process, the theory explains, the individual alleviates intolerable guilt feelings stemming from unconscious and poorly sublimated strivings.

For psychoanalytic theory,

> crime . . . represents a behavioural violation of one or more social norms. Since the cognition of and conformity to social norms are resultants of the socialization process, it follows that the individual who engages in a pattern of criminal behaviour has, in some sense, been defectively socialized or that the norms demanding his conformity are themselves, in some sense, defective. (Feldman, 1964:435)

What the above implies is that society imposes restrictions on the instinctual impulses of an individual. Such impulses are part of the biological make-up of the individual and are essentially antisocial in nature, consisting of the aggressive, destructive and sexual instinct. Individuals must, therefore, reach a psychic balance if they are to retain their normality and adaptation to the environment. In a sense, original impulses (associated with the id), the mechanisms of adjustment (associated with the ego) and the internalisation of group norms (associated with the superego) must be negotiated in order to achieve a 'balance of power'. However, such a balance occurs only in conjunction with the amount of gratification and enforced renunciations individuals experience. Feldman (1964:436) summarises this in these terms:

> Combining now the principle of motivational functionalism and the socialization schema of ego psychology, the basic aetiological formula of psychoanalytic criminology becomes apparent: it simply states that criminality is undertaken as a means of maintaining psychic balance or as an effort to rectify a psychic balance which has been disrupted.

An example of such an imbalance is when offenders are deemed to have gaps in their superego ('superego lacunae'). The offenders' normative orientation, that is to say their 'conscience' (the inner policeman), is undeveloped or defective. These gaps result from the unconscious permissiveness of parental figures who are themselves ambivalent about the acceptance of the norms which prohibit antisocial or criminal acts. It also implies that crime may be the outcome of the internalisation of defective norms which implicates an interaction of biology and environment.

The psychological, biological and genetic theories have useful contributions to make to our understanding of crime. This is particularly relevant to atypical violent crime which, when it happens, touches the conscience of a nation (as in the case of mass murders, such as the Frederick West case, and extreme violent behaviour by young children against other children, for example the James Bulger case). In such cases, these theories have a stronger, higher and more credible relevance and profile to sustain than other theories which are mainly concerned with the more typical sort of crimes associated with this society, namely theft and property offences (including car crime).

The main problem with the psychoanalytic approach is that it is methodologically suspect, as it is difficult to put it to the test: it is difficult to falsify the above assertions as they are deeply embedded in the psyches of individuals. These are not observable and quantifiable characteristics. The approach, as well as most other psychological theories, suffers from the very fact that its premise for the explanation of the criminal act lies in the personality of the offender and other factors appear to be secondary or peripheral. Similarly, biological and genetic explanations of crime emphasise that there is always something which is different in those individuals than in law-abiding citizens. However, this is far from the truth: a considerable amount of research contradicts the view that there is anything intrinsically different between the majority of those who commit criminal acts and those who do not. The most serious flaw in this type of explanation is the absence of any real understanding or acknowledgement that crime, any crime, may not be inherent in the act but is socially constructed. This refers to the type of problems discussed in regard to what is 'crime' in an earlier section of this chapter, and the fact that what is criminal is what the law says it is. One is not denying the reality and severity of the act. The act itself, though, is meaningless if it is not defined, in particular contexts and circumstances, to be criminal. As laws are enacted by individuals, they cannot be anything else but social evaluations of specific social events. It is the evaluation of an act within a social context which makes it criminal or not criminal and not necessarily the personality or biology of an individual. For instance, one state can wage war on another and violence is rewarded with notions of 'bravery', 'courage', 'loyalty' or 'service to one's country'. Those who survive are often celebrated as the 'returning heroes' of a 'proud people'. In a similar but different context, a boxer is permitted to inflict permanent injury on another or even cause death in the course of a fight for a title. In neither case is the loss of life or injury deemed criminal. But if the same returning soldiers engage in a fight outside a public house and inflict injury on each other, that is criminal; if the same boxer uses his skills to knock out someone for shouting abusive remarks, he is deemed to have committed a violent and criminal act. The point here is that such theories do not wish to engage with the grey areas of social life and the social evaluations which go with such experiences; instead they focus on chosen acts which are defined as criminal without questioning the contradictions. Crudely, in the above examples the same individuals appear to be normal in one context, and criminal (or abnormal) in another. In one instance, people are seen as efficient 'fighting machines' and on completion of the task they are decorated for bravery or rewarded with money, glory and titles. In the second instance, the *same* people but in a *different* context are deemed to be extremely violent and dangerous.

Biological and psychological theories are by and large deterministic and reductionist. In their simplest form, individuals have a propensity to be criminal because of those internal and external social factors which make them commit crimes. Individuals are seen as passive and in some sense hapless unless their personality or genetic make-up is altered. This raises serious ethical and moral questions about individual rights and duties. As with economic explanations, they appear to concentrate on the more visible types of crime and it is highly unlikely that such explanations are readily employed to explain the crimes of the powerful. It would be interesting to see a biological, genetic or psychological analysis (a most unlikely event) of the many cases of embezzlement, corporate crime, misapplication of pension funds, bribery of politicians or tax frauds which have bedevilled the socioeconomic and political context of Britain in the 1980s and 1990s. Such an analysis, if applied, would put blame on the biosocial and psychobiological 'defects' of politicians, managing directors of large corporations and media moguls – a legitimate, albeit improbable interpretation.

In contrast to the biological, genetic and psychological theories, *sociological theories* devote most of their attention to the social environment and the nature of social relationships and arrangements. As there are many diverse views on the subject (see Downes and Rock, 1988; Smith, 1995; Williams, 1994), we will offer a few illustrative cases.

One strand (a collection of diverse writings including learning in association with others, cultural influences, social disorganisation and conformity) of sociological theory is referred to as *control theory* (Hirschi, 1969, 1979, 1986; Matza, 1964). Basically, this suggests that inadequate controls are the major reason for crime and social problems in general.

A good example of such an explanation is *social disorganisation*. Crime is seen as a product of lack of social cohesion (e.g. the 'slum'). It is preoccupied with a general breakdown of social controls, isolation and alienation of individuals, and lack of parental control over children: low standards of childcare and a lack of emotional stability in the home. In its basic form, social disorganisation implies a decrease in the influence of existing social rules of behaviour on the individual members of social groups. Conversely, as it is the social environment which is failing individuals (i.e. the environment, as it lacks appropriate controls, is pathologically disorganised), crime may be seen as a 'normal' response to the pathological aspects of the environment. In other words, change the environment and you may gradually change individuals through association with norms and values which are conducive to acceptable behaviour.

Social disorganisation theory's emphasis on the 'normality' of crime in certain neighbourhoods or geographical areas; its point that local characteristics provide a natural milieu in which criminal values emerge and persist; and the realisation it offers that the majority of criminal acts are committed in the company of others (i.e. it is a group enterprise), must be considered as important contributions to understanding crime and debates about methods of intervention. However, it takes for granted that certain values are preferable over others and it smacks of double standards: it concentrates on 'disorganisation' and questions the norms and values missing from that social context, and assumes that everything about traditional or mainstream values is fine and beyond any doubt. So it imposes a set of values which are taken for granted without either close examining or questioning of their relevance or appropriateness. In addition, by designating relationships as disorganised, it denies the fact that to exist at that level there must be some very well defined and organised features or relationships involved. That is exactly where the irony lies. Even the most violent criminal gang is an organised social group, exhibiting refined features of structures and processes which define tasks and roles, rights and duties and normative expectations. Finally, explaining crime and other social problems by resort to social disorganisation theory can be both descriptive and tautological (Downes, 1966): social disorganisation causes crime and crime causes social disorganisation.

Control theory in general is underpinned by processes of socialisation that have gone wrong or which are weak in their maintenance of control over individuals. Some people are able to form proper attachments to the right people and objects (parents, schools, values). They develop a conscience which guides them through life. Others, who are less fortunate, experience the opposite. They form poor attachments and commitments to the right norms and values; or their social milieu is characterised by norms and values that are weak and in conflict with mainstream norms and values. Their actions which follow, therefore, are antithetical to conventional expectations about appropriate behaviour.

In sum, as Smith (1995:39–40) puts it:

> The fundamental complaint about control theory is that . . . it assumes (in extreme versions at least) that we would all be deviant if we dared, with no other motivation than the gratification of our appetites; and that this is the likely outcome if our attachment to others is weak or broken. People are presented as having no internalised sense of values or morality independent of their concern for the good opinion of others. It suggests, implausibly, that we refrain from committing crimes out of fear of losing this good opinion, or in some versions, out of fear of punishment.

Nonetheless, despite these weaknesses, control theory has exercised a formidable hold on policy. Some of the inner city regeneration projects, wars against poverty, neighbourhood schemes, and community work projects (to recreate the lost 'community spirit') have much to do with control theory.

Another set of sociological writings which are normally put together, despite differences in emphasis, to create a competing explanation for criminal acts is what is commonly known as *strain theory*. This considers relations within a given cultural context and social structure. Basically, these sociologists view crime and deviance as socially induced (strain) arising out of unequal access to opportunities. A particular theme of this theory is the concept of *anomie* (Durkheim, 1933, 1970). For Durkheim the term was, in the main, a description of extreme situations of normlessness: that is to say, social conditions where no clear-cut guides to behaviour exist and where previous solutions to problems are rendered inappropriate by social change. Anomie arises when the collective order is disrupted by people's natural (hence biological) aspirations to fulfil higher (personal, egoistic) goals. For Durkheim crime was an inevitable aspect of social relations and he considered it a 'normal' feature of society. Indeed he suggested that, though improbable, a 'society of saints' would be a very unwelcome and oppressive regime. Merton (1957), though accepting Durkheim's thesis, goes a step further by reformulating the concept to imply a friction or disjunction between culturally defined goals and the institutional (social structural) means of achieving them. In so doing, Merton expressed himself as a 'cautious rebel' (Taylor et al., 1973): he was making a cautious statement about unequal access (structural means) to success (cultural goal) in American society. His main concern was to account for the differential distribution of crime rates amongst different social groups. He suggested that societies (American society in his formulation) have dominant goals which all citizens are expected or encouraged to seek and achieve. The notion of the 'American dream', implying personal financial security and success and an affluent and influential social status, captures Merton's idea of the dominant cultural goal. As there is, therefore, a dominant goal, there are also legitimate means (socially and legally defined and approved) which engender access to that success. However, Merton argues that whilst the goals are in abundance, the means are in short supply: legitimate access is restricted to a few. The disjunction causes strain in the system. While the cultural prescriptions are still relevant the legitimate means are blocked by the social structure. As a result the pressure to deviate from the legitimate means and employ illicit means to achieve material success and social rewards is strongest amongst economically and socially disadvantaged groups. This explains why such social groups are over-represented in official statistics and appear to commit more criminal acts.

Merton developed a typology of adaptations (i.e. solutions) for achieving the dominant goal or resolving the conflict which arises from a disjunction between goals and means. Those who are able to achieve the desired goal by legitimate means remain within the mainstream; thus they manage to remain faithful to the rules and normative aspirations. They are the 'conformists'. Others aspire to the goal but have no access to the means. For that, they 'innovate';

that is to say, they use illicit means to achieve the desired outcomes. But there are also those who are not particularly impressed with the goals, nor with the means, and want to change the system. These engage in 'rebellion' and call for a deconstruction and reconstruction of society. However, there are also others who give up both the goals and the means and retreat to more individual instrumental adjustments (e.g. drug-taking, mental illness). There are others too who abandon all hope for success and lose all interest in the means and, therefore, apathy sets in. These are the 'ritualists' who are uninterested in everything and routinely 'play the game'.

Anomie theory has a distinct contribution to make to sociological theory in general and policy in particular. Many postwar policies on crime and poverty in the USA and in Britain have or bear the ideological assumptions of anomie. But as Taylor et al. (1973) have succinctly argued, there are serious problems with anomie too. In particular, it is extremely difficult to conceive of a society where anyone totally 'conforms'. As argued earlier, there is far more crime in a society than official statistics normally show. Anomie theory accepts, without criticism, official crime rates as a true reflection of the incidence of illicit behaviour at any given time. Crime and deviance are far more widespread than that and include crimes of the powerful which, as argued earlier, remain camouflaged or if exposed receive limited attention. Anomie theory, therefore, has been accused of explaining too much 'proletarian criminality' and too little 'bourgeois criminality' (Taylor et al., 1973). In regard to the choices people make, that is to say, the typology of adaptations, they are not clearly explained. One does not know what makes individuals choose one adaptation or another or why not all adaptations at one and the same time. Individually, these adaptations have their own problems too. For example it is not entirely correct to suggest that 'drug misuse' is a retreat from society. In fact, drug misuse is far more socially widespread than is normally assumed and many of those who are seen to be conformists due to their status and respectability (for example the medical profession) may be actively engaging in their normal aspirations while at the same time engaging in serious drug misuse. Furthermore, as has nowadays been recognised, drug misuse may not be a peripheral and contra-cultural lifestyle but one which is deeply ingrained in the social structure of the formal economy (see Ruggiero and Vass, 1992).

As in the case of psychological theories, anomie theory treats the choice (e.g. criminal act) as an abrupt change, a leap from a state of normality to a state of strain and consequently anomie. It omits much reference to social interaction and the existence of reference groups which may encourage or discourage illicit activity.

Whilst Merton considered anomie, and adaptations to that social condition, as an individual concern, others have suggested that illicit activity is better understood as a group activity. Thus Cohen (1955) argued that anomie is useful in explaining some adult crime (as it may be utilitarian in character) but fails to explain the non-utilitarian nature of much of *subcultural* delinquency. Following a similar line of argument to Merton (in relation to the effects of the social structure on criminal activity), Cohen explained the emergence of the subculture of the 'delinquent gang' as a result of a rift between middle-class dominant values and working-class values. As working-class youth are alienated from dominant values they are drawn together by common hostilities. As the subculture which is formed is in direct opposition to the middle-class dominant values, its own natural aspirations are guided by opposition to social control agencies (police, social workers, probation officers). It is characterised by destructiveness, malice towards objects or property and negativism; overall it is a 'hedonistic' culture.

In another reformulation of Merton's anomie, Cloward and Ohlin (1960) made further refinements by connecting the original formulation to Sutherland's notion of 'differential association' (Sutherland and Cressey, 1966) which focuses on the learning process and the transmission of criminal and deviant lifestyles. They argued that criminal (like 'normal' behaviour) is part of a collaborative social activity which gives meaning to individual actions. Individuals achieve success via 'illegitimate opportunities' which are supported and taught by a 'criminal culture' which provides, in contrast to mainstream culture, its own type of lifestyles and opportunities for achievement.

Subcultural theory, like anomie, underestimates the great diversities that exist in a society and between subcultures. These original formulations tend to focus on working-class men or boys and there is a distinct absence of any clear reference to women or girls. They do not explain why some working-class youths or adults become members of a subculture whose main theme is to challenge the legitimacy of the middle-class dominant value whilst others, in similar socioeconomic circumstances, choose to remain 'loyal' to legitimate opportunities even though they may recognise their limited chances for access to shared goals. As Williams (1994:311) also points out, these explanations 'provide no convincing basis to account for the fact that many of the youths tend to reform or stop committing criminal acts at the end of their teens and the onset of adulthood'.

With the progressive development of sociological analyses of crime and deviant behaviour it is now recognised that the same social structures and value systems which give rise to socially approved behaviour and action, can also give rise to socially disapproved ones. It is also recognised that the appraisals reached by judges of such behaviour may reflect the 'world views' of the judges. In other words, crime and its *social control* are seen to be interconnected, leading to significant social consequences. One theoretical perspective which has done much to bring forward this connection and argue that social control is as important a focus of study as criminal acts are, is a particular brand of symbolic interactionism commonly but incorrectly known as *labelling theory*. Unfortunately the use of the term 'labelling' (with its implied consequences of stigma) has taken attention away from the most important foci and contributions of interactionism to the study of crime and focused attention on the least original idea about the use and application of labels in the process of criminalising behaviour. For that matter, to understand the nature of 'labelling theory' and its approach to crime and deviance, one needs to identify its theoretical roots and how those roots have allowed 'labelling theory' to develop into a distinct perspective of crime and deviance.

Labelling theory can be traced back to one of the most important theoretical influences in American sociology and social psychology: symbolic interactionism (see, for instance, Lindesmith and Strauss, 1968; Rose, 1962; Stone and Farberman, 1971). Symbolic interactionism emerged in an unsystematised form from the philosophy of George Herbert Mead, the writings of Charles Horton Cooley, and the ecological studies of Park, Burgess and Faris. A systematised version was provided by Blumer (1969:79), who captured its essence thus:

> The term symbolic interaction refers to the peculiar and distinctive characters of interaction as it takes place between human beings. The peculiarity consists in the fact that human beings interpret or 'define' each other's actions instead of merely reacting to each other's actions. . . . This response . . . is based on the meaning which they attach to such actions. Thus, human interaction is mediated by the use of symbols, by interpretation, or by ascertaining the meaning of one another's actions.

From Blumer's work, symbolic interactionism is characterised as having three foci (Plummer, 1975):

- the social world as a subjective symbolic reality. This focuses on the meanings and the understanding of the ways in which the world is socially constructed;
- the social world as interactive and interrelated. This requires the study of the actor in conjunction with others;

- the social world as a process. This directs the study of social life as constantly changing, with new meanings emerging.

The above foci are central to labelling theory: 'how attitudes about the label become socially meaningful, how they are brought into definitions of varying situations, how they affect the selves of the actors involved and how they change the structure and course of future behaviour among them' (Ericson, 1975:65–6).

Building on symbolic interactionism's major concerns, crime and deviance can be conceptualised in a similar manner (see Plummer, 1975). In the first instance, crime and deviance can be seen as *interaction*. That is to say, labelling theory views crime and deviance as a transactional process, the result of interaction between those who commit an act and those who respond to it. The crucial variable in defining something as illicit or deviant is not the act but the social reaction to it. Crime and deviance are what people decide they are. There is the objective aspect of the act but it will have no consequences unless it is deemed to be criminal (Cohen, 1967). One cannot understand crime by merely looking at the person or the act; one has to consider the reactions of an audience, for it is the type of reaction and the meanings attached to that act which will determine its status. A much quoted passage from Becker (1963:9) captures the essence of how labelling theory sees crime and deviance as inter-action: 'social groups create deviance by making the rules whose infraction constitutes deviance and by applying those rules to particular people and labelling them as outsiders'.

Equally, labelling theory, in the tradition of symbolic interaction-ism, focuses on the collective definitions of an act or phenomenon and on how the process of interpreting the actions of each other leads to a collective act (Ericson, 1975:33). This is well demonstrated by Lemert (1967), who suggests that labelling is the study of 'how deviant acts are symbolically attached to persons and the effective consequences of such attachment for subsequent deviations'. In other words, what labelling theory asserts is that once an act has been defined as criminal or deviant there are both direct conse-quences (e.g. someone is regarded and treated as a criminal) and latent consequences (i.e. once treated as criminal and given, say, his 'just deserts', the individual experiences stigma, rejection and inevit-ably self-reaction leading to changes in his behaviour).

In contrast to sociological theories which consider the social structure and broader concerns, labelling theory concentrates on the 'local dramas', that is micro-sociological concerns and the defi-nitions of the situation. In view of that, when one studies crime in terms of the interaction between those who commit an act and those who react to it one discovers that there is nothing absolute about the interpretations of the situation. That is to say, crime is *subjectively problematic*. So-called 'facts', therefore, are only relevant to a particular time, with particular people in particular social contexts. Acts of crime, in other words, are relative to time, individuals, groups and situations. What may be criminal or deviant now may not be so in future. Symbols, meanings and typifications do not remain static. They are changeable and negotiable.

As can be observed, the notion that nothing is static or absolute implies that interactions have another characteristic. They are dynamic and changing. This means that crime can only be understood as a *process*: 'constantly changing states reflecting complex interaction processes' (Schur, 1969:8). Events have a history, or a 'career'. As Plummer (1975:28) writes, 'Deviancy arises against a backdrop of perpetual change.'

In a nutshell, labelling theory prefers to consider the actions and reactions of individuals in the context of social interaction, the definitions of the situation and how meanings (e.g. that something is criminal) arise out of that interaction. It suggests that studying the rules of the situation (social control) and those who define, administer and enforce those rules (social control agencies) is far more profitable in understanding crime and deviance than focusing on the act itself. Although the act is not denied, labelling theory suggests that it may not be the significant factor which may or may not establish it as criminal or an unacceptable form of action. Furthermore, contrary to previous theories, labelling theory moves the study of crime away from taken for granted views (e.g. that we all know what crime is) and suggests that life events go through stages of development: they are dynamic, blurred and negotiable.

Labelling theory has been subjected to considerable criticism (see Taylor et al. 1973, for a review) particularly because of its insistence that attention should move away from the act to those who define the act as criminal. This criticism is somewhat exaggerated and as said earlier the misconception that 'labelling theory' only refers to one thing – the attachment of 'labels' to other people, stigmatising them for life – has probably done much to encourage misunderstanding of what this brand of symbolic interactionism has to offer to the study of crime. It is true that if one concentrates too much on labels and reactions, diminishing the reality of the harm of the act as though it is all in the mind, there is a real danger of making everything appear relative. As Plummer (1975:25) recognises: 'While the relativising of deviance has a number of important and valuable contributions to make, the enterprise is not without its dangers. Most especially, it can send one hurtling into the relativist collapse by which it becomes possible to argue that anything is deviant and anything goes.'

Another major criticism levelled against the theory is that by focusing on social interaction and thus micro-situational experiences it fails to deal with macro-structural issues. In other words, it becomes critical of local officialdom but leaves the real power relationships (the 'higher-ups') unscathed (Taylor et al., 1973). In fairness, the very theoretical position which this perspective adopts (that of symbolic interactionism) cannot be anything but micro-sociological. And as Rock (1973:14–15) has suggested, 'Even if it is assumed that large-scale social structures have a logic and organisation . . . attempts to predict their development may falter unless they employ material derived from the micro-sociological plane'. Given that the theory considers that social reactions are a particularly important factor in the social construction of criminal acts, in policy terms it adopts a 'hands-off' approach or preaches tolerance. Attempts to 'destructure' the prison establishment by a policy of diverting offenders to community penalties and shielding juvenile delinquents from the criminal justice system (e.g. police cautioning) have, in part, their roots in this perspective.

Although the theories covered thus far have raised various questions about unequal access to life chances, the role of administrators and law enforcers, none has directed its attention to the role of the state in the process of managing and controlling its citizens. *Conflict theory* and *critical criminology* emphasise the role of the state in maintaining order and unequal power relationships. The conflict approach to crime emerged as a conception of society in terms of competing definitions of reality held by diverse groups in society. People and groups may share some common values (partial consensus) but they also have marked differences in normative orientation and power. Inevitably there is conflict between social groups, and social order is a temporary and passing phase until conflict emerges again which leads to change. These theories see the powerful gaining control of the legal order and using that order to increase their hold on power. Although unconnected with conflict theorists, the political writer Schattscheider, in making an observation about the claim that 'pluralist states' are democratic, said: 'the flaw in the pluralist heaven is that the heavenly chorus sings with a strong upper-class accent'. The observation goes a long way to capture the gist of the conflict theorists' main concern.

If the powerful use the law to further their interests it means that the law is used as an instrument of state control. Criminality is essentially a 'metaphor': in reality it is a power relationship (an authority versus subject conflict). However, the way in which the authority/subject relationship develops depends on who is involved in the relationship. Laws affect people with different social economic and political characteristics differently. Criminality constitutes a status which is applied by others who have the power to do so and higher interests to sustain (Turk, 1969). 'Crime' then is a political act. It is constructed by the enactment of laws by the powerful. The law is accepted by the rest as a legitimate affair. Once it is accepted and the powerless summit to the authority of the law, the powerful are bestowed with the right to pursue and promote their class interests (Quinney, 1970). Conversely, crime is a conscious way of resisting and changing that culture. Crime and deviance are normal responses to the type of social and political structures which characterise unequal societies. Removing such inequalities and recognising human diversity would render the existence of a legally oppressive system unnecessary (Taylor et al., 1973, 1975). In other words, the state will no longer have to defend itself by creating laws to patch up the pathologies it has created by its own system (Quinney, 1974).

Conflict and critical criminologists are influenced by Marx and Engels. They place the study and understanding of crime in its political context, that is the political economy. Along with Marxists such as Lukacs and Lenin these criminologists use their position as intellectuals to define reality to the underdog, to create the correct class consciousness and rescue the masses from false consciousness (Taylor et al., 1973). However, the politicisation of crime incorporates other strands of theory, particularly aspects of symbolic interactionism. Although its focus is on the political economy and therefore on broader social structures within which social relationships take place, its definition of crime as a socially constructed power relationship – that all human behaviour is normal as opposed to pathological unless it goes through a process of typification and designation as criminal and deviant – is an essential focus of interactionism, as pointed out earlier in the chapter.

The politicisation of crime, though heralded as a new and revitalised look at the social construction of crime in the early 1970s, is actually very old and few people have realised this. The idea that crime is a social evaluation leading to social and state controls established by the powerful to contain others and that the law is a means to that end can be traced back well before the writings of such theorists or their founding 'fathers', Marx, Engels and Bonger, and the writings of Charles Horton Cooley, George Herbert Mead, W.I. Thomas, Robert E. Park, Ernest Burgess, William Ogburn and Phil Hauser, who are associated with the birth of interactionism. Indeed some of the basic tenets of interactionism in combination with critical criminology can be found in the debates between philosopher and students in the *agora* in ancient Greece dating from about 410 BC. In Plato's *Republic* (Plato, 1955) a student of Socrates, Thrasymachus (who constantly agitated his teacher by rejecting the 'official' definitions of social and moral issues; in modern Greek his name is associated with *thrasis*, meaning someone who is extremely rude), questioned Socrates' argument that laws are enacted to protect most citizens' interests and to draw acceptable boundaries between right and wrong. Thrasymachus argued that it does not matter whether you refer to states which are characterised by 'tyranny' or 'democracy'. In each state, he said, 'power is in the hands of the ruling class' (Plato, 1955:66). Thrasymachus went on to explain his assertion in words which could easily have been 'lifted' from the writings of interactionists, conflict and critical criminologists:

> *Each ruling class makes laws that are in its own interest*, a democracy democratic laws, a tyranny tyrannical ones and so on; and in making these laws they define as 'right' for their subjects what is in the interests of themselves, the rulers, and *if anyone breaks their laws he is punished as a 'wrong-doer'*. (Plato, 1955:66; emphasis added)

As with all other theories, conflict and critical criminology adds new knowledge to the 'puzzle' called crime by pointing out another social dimension to engendering state control and keeping society orderly. But conflict and critical criminology suffers from a number of weaknesses – for example, the idea that social order and the resultant consensus is the result of a process of 'mystification' (Taylor et al., 1973); a reality created by the powerful (Taylor et al., 1975); and that crime is merely the violation of ruling-class legitimacy is rather far-fetched. Although there is an attractive ring to the idea, if not some truth in it, and for many people this may create some sort of affinity with their personal values which criticise inequality and injustice, it is difficult to know who exactly that 'ruling class' is. It is folly to believe that the powerful and the ruling class are one and the same socially identifiable and cohesive group. There is no attempt to differentiate between elites and to discuss such elites and power groups as competing enterprises. They are presented as a homogeneous group that usually pulls the strings. Such a view does not reflect the real world of diversity, competing perspectives and conflicts of interest: the powerful and the rich are often sharply in competition for economic and political power, and the poor are most of the time in competition amongst themselves rather than with the higher-ups. It is unrealistic to believe that all the rich share the same values and interests or that all the poor work together against the common enemy: the rich, powerful and the state. Indeed, one can argue that in the poorer areas of any given city it is the horizontal competition and conflict (e.g. much crime is directed by the poor against the poor), not vertical conflict (crimes against the powerful) which is the norm.

Furthermore, it is difficult to relate much of crime to the notion that it is political resistance against the powerful. It is questionable whether individuals who commit crimes impute a political meaning to their acts: 'I steal from you because that is my attempt to challenge the existing social and political order'; 'As a man, I commit crimes against women because I want to draw attention to the inequalities which exist in this society and the role of masculinity in this unequal relationship'. It is also questionable whether stealing someone's jewels, antiques, money or other possessions is likely to create a tremor, a social earthquake, which will shake the social order and force it to collapse to be replaced with something new.

A third criticism is that such theorists tend to underestimate the benefits accrued for the poorer and more powerless groups in society as a result of laws and changes in the laws. It is not acceptable simply to argue that such groups are mystified and cajoled into accepting the legitimacy of the social order created by the power elites. In addition, once laws are enacted they can also be used, as they have been (although not too often) to deal with crimes of the powerful, and indeed against the very people who have enacted them. In a similar vein, it is implausible to suggest that from the underdog's point of view the commission of a criminal act is symbolic of efforts to challenge the hegemony of the power elite, when in fact much white-collar crime (and crimes of the powerful in general) is committed and directed by such power elites against other power elites. It is a contradiction in terms. First the theory ignores these types of crime as they do not fit well into its schema, and secondly it is difficult to envisage the same power elites which exercise control over others conspiring behind the scenes to bring down their own oligarchy.

A last illustration of the flaws in such an approach is the fact that in trying to politicise crime, the theory, by implication, ignores or underestimates the harm done by crime to *victims* (who, as said earlier, are mainly 'powerless' people too). If crime is a political challenge to the authority of the ruling class, then implicitly victims of crime are rejected or written off as an unfortunate but unavoidable aspect of the social struggle against 'tyranny'. It is almost as though Napoleon's dictum that 'you cannot make an omelette without breaking eggs' fits well with this theory. The problem is that the broken eggs are real people living in the reality of crime (irrespective of definitions) and the fear of crime.

It was left to other theorists – particularly a 'revisionist' group of criminologists who had in the past espoused the merits of critical or radical criminology – to attempt to consider the plight of victims in the context of both micro- and macro-level relationships which define, measure, react, shape and control crime. This is what is known as *realist criminology*. Although there are important differences between right realism (see Wilson, 1985) and left realism (see, for instance, Matthews and Young, 1992; Young and Matthews, 1992) and it is inappropriate to place them in one category (see Williams, 1994), in the main, at least in the British context, they are keen to address just about every aspect of crime and prevention: offenders, victims, crime rates, fear of crime, social control agencies, public perceptions and reactions among others. In contrast to earlier theory, realist criminologists recognise that crime inflicts harm on property and people and creates further pockets of deprivation and exclusion from normal social relationships. In addition to the actual harm, it creates fear and thus has latent effects too. They recognise that victimisation is far more horizontal in character than vertical: that it takes place in the poorer and most socially and economically deprived neighbourhoods which are least able either to resist crime or to cope with its destructive effects. In contrast, the effects of crime on more affluent people or neighbourhoods may have similar harmful effects but such social groups or neighbourhoods can be afforded better services (e.g. police support) and can draw on their affluence to cope with economic and psychological consequences of crime. In other words, they have the social and economic resources to deal with crime far better than their poor counterparts. In essence, realist criminologists distinguish between different people (e.g. men and women, young and older people) and social contexts in terms of how they experience and cope with crime.

Left realists (Matthews and Young, 1992; Young and Matthews, 1992) encompass diverse causes and explanations for crime but are clear as to what they believe to be the most influential variable in either increasing or decreasing crime: social and economic deprivation, with a particular emphasis on the effects of relative deprivation. This is the normative orientation which defines not what people need in an absolute sense but what they think they *should* have in order to feel they are sharing and achieving, with the rest of the population, the same lofty goals. This explains the reason why crime is rising at times of so-called affluence – because there is injustice: people's relative expectations are heightened but few can reach the level of existence which can allow them to satisfy their relative needs. These people are mainly to be found in the mass of the unemployed, minority ethnic groups or other marginalised groups. Inevitably, crime rates will reflect an over-representation of offenders from such groups as they are striving to use illicit methods to satisfy their relative needs. The same illicit methods used as means to achieve more social and material success are also employed by affluent individuals in their search to satisfy even higher goals. As higher goals are reached, relative deprivation creates new depths, and so on.

In many ways, realist criminology has come full circle by incorporating a number of features from other theories, particularly restoring the earlier attraction of anomie theory in the Mertonian sense. Simply, we are back to a disjunction between normative orientation and social structure. The first prescribes the normative goals (e.g. 'self-interest', 'richness', 'material possessions') and the second provides the means. Unfortunately, as opportunities are few, the desire to share others' success leads to crime. 'Greed', therefore, as mentioned earlier, resurfaces as a corrupting element in the process of feeling relatively deprived. Greed has no bounds: it applies to both rich and poor. In consequence, realist criminologists view the reduction of control of crime as a complex network of activities which involve not only policing, community and neighbourhood schemes, situational controls, clear policies about victims and so on, but also the incorporation of social policy which restores justice (better housing, equal opportunities in the economy, better education and so on) and decreases feelings of relative deprivation. In all this, there is also the implicit Weberian notion that 'ideas' are as important, if not more important, in generating praxis. Society needs to be guided by notions of social responsibility and solidarity as opposed to individualism, self-help (implying self-interest), competition and divisions.

Other than being a wide assortment of theoretical positions and dispositions, realist criminology is neither new nor particularly sophisticated. It suffers from a measure of naivety, thinking that if one considers all possible or relevant factors, crime becomes more understandable as well as more amenable to control. In particular, realist criminologists' notion that communities can be helped to resist and fight crime through participation in the policing of their own areas, or in closer collaboration with formal policing agencies, or in closer work with victims is ambitious (see for instance, Smith, 1995:92–110; Pearson et al., 1992). It ignores the diversities existing in any single neighbourhood and the problems of maintaining the community spirit in a cohesive and consistent way over a long period of time. Any community worker who has attempted to enlist the support of the 'community' to address social issues affecting their lives will testify to the intractable problems faced when trying to establish coalitions amongst diverse interests (Vass, 1990:73–6); and how problematic indeed it is to attempt to enlist the support of diverse agencies (Broad, 1996) in crime prevention (Gilling, 1996).

Finally, it is important to state that much of criminology and discussions on crime and its causes is dominated by 'masculinity'. Women have either been treated as peripheral to concerns about crime, or if they have been the focus of study it is because masculine criminology has treated them as an aberration which needed explanation. *Feminist criminology* has attempted to redress the imbalance (see, for example, Buckley, 1996; Campbell, 1984; Cornwall and Lindisfane, 1994; Carlen, 1988; Dobash and Dobash, 1980; Gelsthorpe, 1989; Gelsthorpe and Morris, 1990; Heidensohn, 1985; Messerschmidt, 1993; Simon, 1975; Smart, 1989).

The literature which has been generated by feminist criminology, and its effects on criminology, is extensive and readers ought to familiarise themselves with the debates and contributions (see Smith, 1995; Williams, 1994 for detailed reviews). David Smith's (1995:113) interpretation of the contribution of feminist criminology is worth reproducing here:

> feminist writing has enriched the discipline in four main ways. First, it has shown that much previous criminology neglected the offending of women almost entirely; it was simply assumed that when discussing offenders one was discussing males. Alternatively, female offenders were discussed in a way which emphasised individual abnormality and underplayed the importance of social factors in understanding their offending; even when sociological approaches had become dominant in criminology as a whole, female offending was still generally 'explained' in terms of biological or psychological abnormality. Secondly, feminist writing has called attention to the treatment of females within the criminal justice system. . . . Thirdly, feminism has opened out a new area of study in stressing the importance of previously 'hidden' forms of crime such as domestic violence and sexual abuse within the supposed safety of the home . . . and how victims, or survivors, can best be supported. . . . Finally . . . feminist writing has focused attention on the highly gendered nature of criminal activity, asking both why females commit so few offences and why males commit so many . . . [i.e.] what is it about masculinity which makes being male the best predictor of offending?

A number of theories were discussed in this section. Explanations of crime are varied and no single, general theory exists that captures in any satisfactory way the complexity of this particular aspect of social relationships. Although these and other explanations can be conveniently separated into, say, distinct economic, biological, psychological and sociological categories, this is somewhat arbitrary.

There is always an interplay of the various explanations and the distinctions should be considered as blurred. Nonetheless, each approach has and offers its own relevant knowledge and leads to particular types of intervention and ways of working with offenders.

*The organisation of the criminal justice system*
Another important area which is relevant to competent work is knowledge about the workings of the constituent parts of the criminal justice system. Without an appreciation of the social context of work with offenders it is not possible to understand policy matters, power relationships and accountability.

**The higher echelons**    The Home Secretary is responsible for policy and is answerable to Parliament, though political theorists have always raised questions about this ideal model of the democratic process. They suggest that in reality, due to the 'prime ministerial government' in this country and prime ministerial patronage together with the inner circle of ministerial government, it is the government that dictates to Parliament and the people. Nonetheless, in theory at least, the minister is accountable to the 'people's representatives'.

The Home Secretary and government colleagues in general are legally advised by the government's Attorney-General, who is legally qualified and a member of the government. The Attorney-General, assisted by the Solicitor-General, offers legal assistance on points of law, initiates legal action in regard to 'national matters' or the 'public interest' (e.g. when ex-members of the intelligence services publish memoirs, as in the case of the late Peter Wright, which are deemed to be a threat to national security, or when newspapers breach *sub judice* rules). The Attorney-General's duties also include direct advice to the Crown Prosecution Service (CPS). In effect, like the Home Secretary, the Attorney-General is accountable to Parliament for the way in which the CPS operates.

**The probation service**    The Home Secretary sets policy, aims and priorities for the probation service and the standards to which the service works (e.g. Home Office, 1995a; Home Office et al., 1995). The Home Secretary is supported by the Home Office Probation Service Division. Its purpose is:

- to develop and promote Government policy on the supervision of offenders in the community and other aspects of probation practice
- to assist individual probation services to serve the courts and the public in an efficient and effective way through:
    effective and equitable practice

high standards of management
partnership with other statutory and non-statutory organisations.
(Home Office, 1995a:5)

HM Inspectorate of Probation reports to the Home Secretary on aspects of quality. It inspects the performance of the probation service and allied organisations, 'assessing quality and value for money' (Home Office, 1995a:6), and checks that courts, offenders and the public receive effective and efficient service by those working in probation and allied services. In addition, it advises the Home Secretary on policy in regard to probation and other relevant areas.

In England and Wales there are 56 probation committees or boards which are responsible for local management of each service (see Holdaway, 1996). These are local magistrates appointed by the Lord Chancellor's Office, one or more judge from the Crown Court, co-opted members and local authority members. They are responsible for the appointment, remuneration and performance of all staff. As their statutory duties are to ensure the provision of services and that those services are efficient and effective, and they control budgets in regard to expenditure, they are directly accountable to the Home Secretary.

Executive responsibility for the probation services' functions is held by chief officers of probation. They are accountable to the probation committees and their main role and task is management of the service, strategic planning, monitoring and improving service delivery, working within budgets and managing staff and recruitment.

Area services are financed through local authorities, which receive 80 per cent of expenditure from the Home Office. In 1994–95 central government provided a total of £417 million for offender programmes, probation in prisons, probation service expenditure and capital grants and credit approvals. In 1995–96 this was reduced to £412 million, and projections for the next two years estimate expenditure at approximately £424 million per annum (Home Office, 1995b:11).

**The police** Since October 1986, following the introduction of the Crown Prosecution Service (CPS), the police have ceased to act as prosecutors. Nonetheless, the majority of prosecutions in England and Wales are initiated and prepared by the police in the form of laying charges or information against suspects. The police carry out preliminary investigations prior to considering what action to take and thus they provide a screening process which determines who will be prosecuted. As argued earlier, their part in this process defines knowledge about crime, statistics and, in a sense (subject to the CPS's decisions) the number of court cases. In effect they are an agency which is not only actively involved in the prosecution of offenders but also has the power to socially construct crime and reactions to it.

The police and CPS work closely together since they remain the official and legitimate agency which is vested with the powers to investigate the case or evidence further and report such further inquiries back to CPS. Additionally, their close relationship with CPS is governed by the fact that they are, after all, the Crown's main witnesses in cases where CPS recommends prosecution. It is important to emphasise that the police's task is to investigate the commission of a crime and initiate prosecutions. It is up to the CPS to weigh up the evidence and decide whether the case merits continuation in the courts. The actual presentation of the case against a suspect in court is the CPS's role, not the police's.

As in the case of probation services, the police are made up of various forces, which can exhibit serious differences from each other. They are headed by a chief officer (Chief Constable) except the City of London and Metropolitan police forces, which are headed by a Commissioner. The chief officer is responsible for the force's reputation, efficiency and budgetary aspects and for general or specific policy including decisions about commencing investigations and prosecutions of suspects. Each force is directly accountable to a police authority which involves local authority representatives including magistrates. The Home Office retains direct responsibility for the City of London and Metropolitan forces. As Sprack (1995) explains, the police authority's powers to interfere with the day-to-day organisational issues and decisions of police forces are limited. Indeed, 'the police authority should not interfere in operational terms. . . . In particular, they should not interfere with the police discretion on whether or not to commence prosecutions, either by seeking to influence general policy on the kinds of cases in which prosecutions are appropriate or by ordering a prosecution in a particular case' (Sprack, 1995:5).

**The Crown Prosecution Service**   Staff are accountable to the chief crown prosecutors who lead the various geographical areas of the service. There are 31 areas that make up the CPS which 'correspond roughly to the areas of the 43 police forces in England and Wales' (Sprack, 1995:6). Within each area there are barristers or solicitors designated as crown prosecutors, whose task is to conduct criminal proceedings. These crown prosecutors can represent the service in magistrates' courts but not in the Crown Court. Proceedings in the Crown Court are conducted by private barristers hired by the CPS.

The chief crown prosecutors are, in turn, accountable to the Director of Public Prosecutions (DPP) who holds full responsibility for all proceedings, the conduct of proceedings and advice to police forces, and who presents witnesses for the prosecution as directed by the court, and carries out any other functions as requested by the Attorney-General (Sprack, 1995).

**Courts** Matters which may be of importance in deciding what type of court will deal with criminal cases include the age of the offender and whether the offence is triable only on indictment, summarily or either way. Offences which are triable only on indictment (e.g. murder, manslaughter) must be dealt with by the Crown Court. Summary offences, which are deemed to be less serious, are normally dealt with by magistrates' courts. Offences that are triable either way (i.e. on indictment or summarily) can be dealt with by either magistrates or the Crown Court. This depends on whether the accused opts for trial in the Crown Court or the magistrates consider that their powers to deal with the seriousness of the offence are inadequate and thus may refer the case to the Crown Court.

The age of the defendant is crucial in deciding where the case will be tried. Generally, adult offenders (aged 18 or over) are sentenced in the magistrates' court or the Crown Court depending on the seriousness of the offence. Under the Criminal Justice Act 1991, those aged 17 and under are normally dealt with in the youth court though occasionally they may be tried on indictment if the offence is of such a serious nature that the Children and Young Persons Act 1933 section 53(2) is invoked. The type of sentence available for each group (particularly for juveniles aged 10–17) is determined by the age of the offender at the time of conviction and not the time of the commission of the offence.

In the Crown Court there are five types of judge. High Court judges who are normally attached to the Queen's Bench Division (which deals with civil matters beyond the jurisdiction of the county court and appeals on point of law from the magistrates' court) are full-time judges. They may sit in the Crown Court and normally deal with the most serious criminal cases (e.g. class 1 offences such as treason, murder and offences against national security, and class 2 offences such as infanticide, rape and manslaughter). Subject to approval by the Lord Chief Justice, trial for murder may be conducted by a circuit judge whilst class 2 offences can be tried by either a High Court Judge or a circuit judge.

Circuit judges, who are also full-time, are appointed on the Lord

Chancellor's recommendation. Their responsibilities cover both the Crown Court and county courts. They are appointed from barristers with at least ten years' experience or from recorders who have held office for more than three years. Retirement is normally at 72 though they may be allowed to continue in service until the age of 75.

Recorders are normally barristers or solicitors with a minimum of ten years' experience and their appointment by the Lord Chancellor, to sit at the Crown Court, is for a fixed period and on a part-time basis.

Additionally, if there is considerable pressure on the Crown Court and it appears not to be coping with the number of cases, the Lord Chancellor may appoint retired judges (Lord Justices of Appeal, High Court or circuit judges) as deputy circuit judges to assist in the process. Assistant recorders can also be appointed for the same reason from the ranks of barristers or solicitors with a minimum of ten years' experience.

Magistrates, on the other hand, are by and large 'lay justices', that is to say, unpaid men and women who may or may not have any legal training. They are appointed by the Lord Chancellor on the advice of local committees. Although in recent times attempts have been made to appoint magistrates from diverse social and ethnic backgrounds, the majority still represent the wealthy, white, middle-class business and other interests. A minority are paid, full-time 'stipendiary magistrates', qualified lawyers who are formally appointed on the advice of the Lord Chancellor. These come from the ranks of barristers or solicitors with a minimum of seven years' standing.

In view of the fact that the majority of magistrates have no legal training, much authority is vested in the hands of the clerk to the justices who is normally helped by a deputy or assistant. The clerk is normally required to be a barrister or solicitor with at least five years' experience. As Wasik (1993:42, emphasis in original) states:

> Case-law stresses that the clerk's task is to *advise* the magistrates on matters of sentencing law and procedure, and not to *influence* their decision on the facts. In practice, however, this sharp distinction is a rather difficult one to achieve and in some cases, the clerk may have a significant influence upon the bench's sentencing decision.

Finally, proceedings in the youth court are conducted by magistrates who are elected (every three years) to sit on a special youth court panel and who are given specific training in dealing with juveniles. Only this panel of elected members can summarily try juveniles. The youth court must sit with at least two magistrates; no stipendiary magistrate is allowed to sit alone.

Above and beyond those three courts there is the High Court which is made up of three divisions. The Queen's Bench Division deals with appeals from magistrates' courts on point of law and with civil matters which are beyond the powers of the county courts. The Chancery Division is mainly concerned with disputes in regard to taxes and trusts. The Family Division has similar responsibilities to the family proceedings and county courts.

The Court of Appeal comprises two divisions, one (the Criminal Division, headed by the Lord Chief Justice) dealing with cases referred to it on appeal by the Crown Court; and the other (Civil Division, headed by the Master of the Rolls) which deals with appeals from the High and county courts. The Court of Appeal interprets the law and as such its decisions set legal precedents.

The House of Lords is the highest body, and deals with points of law which are regarded to be of extreme public significance. Reference to the House of Lords can take place only with the consent of the Court of Appeal. Its membership consists of five of the most senior Law Lords, and their decision is binding.

*Sentencing and national standards*

This section will concentrate on community penalties (Vass, 1996) or as the law (Criminal Justice Act 1991) and national standards (Home Office et al., 1995) refers to them, 'community sentences' (see also Ward and Ward, 1993). For a wider coverage of sentencing issues, the law and sentencing principles the reader should consult other texts (see Geary, 1994; Sprack, 1995; Wasik, 1993; Wasik and Taylor, 1991).

The range of sentences available to courts is often referred to as the 'tariff', as they represent a 'ladder' of disposals according to their severity. However, it must be stressed that although one can build a convenient ladder with each step (sentencing option) leading to a higher and more severe penalty, courts are not always predictable and the tariff is not always followed in rigid fashion by sentencers. Notwithstanding that qualification, at the bottom of the ladder there are the discharge orders and fines. These are followed by community sentences: probation, community service order, combination order, attendance centre order and curfew order (though the last of these still remains inactivated). At the top of the ladder sit suspended sentences of imprisonment and custody for both adults (imprisonment for anyone aged 21 and over) and juveniles (detention in a young offenders' institution for those aged 15 to 20).

In trying to reach a decision on the appropriate sentence, courts are faced with four questions. First, is the sentence for the offence fixed by law (e.g. murder and high treason)? If so, there is little choice but to follow the rules. Secondly, if not fixed by law, the court must consider what options are available to it in deciding the appropriate sentence and the specific circumstances within which each option can be available (e.g. age of the offender, maximum penalty, pre-sentence reports). Thirdly, there is the seriousness of the offence and 'what level of sentence would properly reflect the seriousness of the offence', although 'It is very difficult to define "seriousness" in the abstract, and no attempt is made to do so in existing sentencing law' (Wasik, 1993:54). Fourthly, are there any mitigating circumstances which need to be taken into account?

In addition to those questions courts as well as other agencies in the criminal justice system must consider how to avoid discrimination 'on the ground of race or sex or any other improper ground' (Criminal Justice Act 1991, section 95).

There is considerable debate about whether sentencing patterns vary according to race but recent findings appear to suggest that when all the intervening variables are taken into account (e.g. nature of the offence, previous convictions) there are no statistically significant differences in the sentencing pattern for black, Asian and white offenders. The higher number of black offenders receiving custodial and longer sentences in comparison to white offenders is more a function of the seriousness of the offences than of race (Hood, 1993). However, the findings also show that black and Asian defendants are less likely to have pre-sentence reports prepared for them by the probation service and where such reports are prepared these offenders are less likely to be recommended for probation (evidence suggests that the same applies to other community penalties: see Vass, 1996).

As regards gender issues, there is clear evidence that there are distinct differences between the way courts deal with men and women. Women are less likely to be given a community service order but are more likely to be given a probation or supervision order, for example. Also, when all age groups are considered for indictable offences, women are more likely to be given a discharge order than men. Women, nonetheless, are found to be less 'criminal' than men (law-breaking is mainly a male 'preoccupation') and their offences are less serious; they also have less serious criminal records (Home Office, 1992).

For a range of penal sanctions, including custodial sentences, available to courts see the summary in Jones et al. (1992) and for greater detail refer to Sprack (1995:229–311) and Wasik (1993:79–363). For a detailed discussion on community sentences see above, and also Home Office et al. (1995) and Ward and Ward (1993). In this section we will summarise the major points about community penalties which should guide the practice of anyone working with offenders, though again it should be strongly emphasised that practitioners must ensure that they familiarise themselves with the full and often complex details of available sanctions. Furthermore, it must be remembered that knowledge, as argued in Chapter 1, is a dynamic process which has a career: it constantly changes. Available sanctions are modified or amended by law, or are discontinued or complemented by new requirements or other penalties and so on. Thus whilst one may currently refer to 'community sentences' under the Criminal Justice Act 1991, in future this may change under new legislation which may extend the present range of community penalties or introduce 'a single integrated sentence incorporating the . . . range of community orders' currently available (Home Office, 1995a:19). Facts about penal sanctions, types, requirements and so forth must not be taken for granted as they may be dated and thus inapplicable. Practitioners must always strive to keep up with changes in the legislation and ensure that they possess all the relevant knowledge about each penalty as it applies to their working environment. Similarly, other than the knowledge of what is available and under what conditions, the practitioner should be familiar with the *procedural* aspects of the supervision of offenders and the application of those sanctions. In sum, the motto of every student and practitioner ought to be: a law is for today, not for tomorrow.

There is much confusion about what exactly 'community penalties', or 'community sentences' or more generally 'non-custodial options' really entail in practice. As pointed out elsewhere they normally refer to a 'wide assortment of tasks and dispositions' which lack clarity (Vass, 1996). In this section 'community sentences' and 'community penalties' will be used interchangeably to refer to the six community orders incorporated within the framework of the Criminal Justice Act 1991: probation, community service, combination, curfew, supervision and attendance centre orders. All, except the supervision order and attendance centre order, are available for all offenders aged 16 or over. The supervision order is available for those aged 10 to 17 years inclusive; and the attendance centre order for anyone aged 10 to 20 years inclusive. In view of the fact that attendance centre orders are not supervised by the probation service or social services departments and are the prerogative of the police; and the curfew order, though introduced by the Criminal Justice Act 1991, is not yet implemented (but see Home Office, 1995a for new intentions), they will not be covered in this chapter and the reader is referred to other sources (for example, Ward and Ward, 1993).

Community penalties developed 'piecemeal over many years. The last substantively new penalty to be introduced was community service [order] in 1973' (Home Office, 1995a:5). The Criminal Justice Act 1991 extended the range of community orders, established them within a common framework and made the probation order for the first time a sentence of the court (rather than in lieu of a sentence). This common framework is guided by the notion of proportionality. It requires that community penalties 'can only be imposed where the relevant offences, taking account of previous offences or failure to respond to previous sentences, are "serious enough" for such a sentence but not "so serious" that only custody is justified' (Home Office, 1995a:6). Community sentences are intended to punish offenders by restricting their liberty but without segregating them from their communities. Certain community penalties (the probation, community service, combination and curfew orders and where certain special requirements are included in a supervision order: see Sprack, 1995:286) can be imposed only if offenders give their consent (though this matter of consent is under review: see Home Office, 1995a).

It is the task of the courts, not the probation officer or other practitioners, to apply the law by imposing community penalties. The role of the social worker or probation officer is to assist the court in its sentencing decisions. One way which enables the court to consider the relevant information before considering the appropriateness of a community penalty is the production of a pre-sentence report (PSR) (for a detailed discussion on PSRs see Smith, 1996). Under the Criminal Justice Act 1991, PSRs, which have replaced the social inquiry reports, are mandatory for the following community penalties:

- a probation order with additional requirements;
- a community service order;
- a combination order;
- a supervision order with specific requirements under the Children and Young Persons Act 1969 section 12 (A, AA, B, C).

However, the Criminal Justice and Public Order Act 1994 has amended the above requirement and courts may use their discretion in deciding whether a PSR is necessary or unnecessary for offenders aged 18 or over. Despite this amendment, the courts are still required to consider all information about the circumstances of the offence, including any aggravating or mitigating factors, that is available to them. Where courts may require a PSR, 'this may include an indication of the expected level of supervision, together with some elements of the content of any particular order which is proposed. Following the National Standards review, an outline supervision plan will become a required feature of a PSR' (Home Office, 1995a:8).

The national standards (Home Office et al., 1995) set out the requirements for preparing PSRs. The basic tenets are thus: a report should be impartial, balanced and factually accurate as far as possible. Its purpose is to provide 'a professional assessment' of the circumstances, nature and causes of an individual's crime and what action is proposed to reduce the likelihood of re-offending. If an offender does not consent to the preparation of a PSR and the court still requires one, the practitioner must strive to produce a report 'using the information available' and explain to the court that the offender was uncooperative. The offender (or those with parental responsibility, as in the case with young offenders) should be given at least two opportunities for the preparation of the report; and 'reasonable' steps should be taken to collect additional information from other sources (in the case of a young offender a school report may be relevant). The attempts to collate information and the sources of information should be made clear in the report. It is also important that the report writer consults with the police with regard to antecedents and relevant circumstances. If an offender is unable to communicate effectively (due to language differences, hearing difficulties or other reasons) it is expected that an 'accredited interpreter' will be used.

There has been a very long debate about how best to present reports (see Smith, 1996). National standards specify a format for good practice. The front sheet which normally contains the individual and personal details of the offender, the court, the court hearing date, and the name of the report writer, should also include a headline paragraph which states: 'This is a pre-sentence report as defined in section 3(5) of the Criminal Justice Act 1991. It has been prepared in accordance with the requirements of the National Standards for pre-sentence reports. This report is a confidential document' (Home Office et al., 1995:8).

The main report should have five major sections: an introduction, a discussion and analysis of the offence, the relevant information about the offender, the risk to the public of re-offending and a conclusion which ties up loose ends and which flows 'logically and directly from the rest of the report' (Home Office et al., 1995:11). For a full statement on the required standards and what information should be covered under each heading, refer to Home Office et al. (1995:8–16; see also Smith, 1996).

Some basic things to remember in preparing reports are as follows:

- The sources of information must always be made clear.
- If an interpreter has been used, this must be indicated.
- The status of the offender (that is to say, is he/she known to the report writer, probation service or social services department?) must be given.
- A balanced picture of the offender (strengths and weaknesses) must be given.
- The report need not, and normally should not, include full details of the offender's criminal history (this is the prosecution's task).
- Information should be limited to what is relevant to sentencing.
- The report should be written in a clear language, free of jargon, be coherent, accurate and concise without grammatical and spelling errors.

In reports presented for the youth court, it is imperative that the writer takes into account the Children and Young Persons Act 1933 section 44 which 'requires the court to have regard for the welfare of the individual. The United Nations Convention on the Rights of the Child, to which the United Kingdom is a signatory, also requires that in all actions concerning children, i.e. those aged below 18 years, in courts of law the best interests of the child shall be the primary consideration' (Home Office et al., 1995:13).

Finally, matters of confidentiality need to be taken into consideration. Reports should not be distributed or disclosed beyond the confines of the case (courts) without the offender's consent. The offender is entitled to be given a copy of the report by the probation service or social services department, and this 'should be read aloud to those who cannot read, or read aloud in translation for those whose first language is not English' (Home Office et al., 1995:14).

A *probation order* may be made on an offender aged 16 years or over. This requires the individual to be under the supervision of the probation service for a period of not less than six months and not more than three years. Additional requirements can be included (Criminal Justice Act 1991, Part II, schedule 1). These may be a residence requirement, a treatment requirement, a probation centre requirement, an 'active' requirement (that is to say, to participate in certain prescribed activities) or a 'negative' requirement (that is to say, the court may prohibit the offender from participating in specified activities).

The objectives of the order are to 'secure the rehabilitation of the offender', to 'protect the public from harm' and to 'prevent the offender from committing further offences'. It is expected that the supervising officer will challenge offenders to accept responsibility for their crimes and their consequences and make 'offenders aware of the impact of the crimes they have committed on victims, the community and themselves' (Home Office et al., 1995:17).

The supervising officer should arrange a meeting with the offender within five working days of the making of the order. The offender should be served with a copy of the order and asked to sign; be issued with instructions stating the required standards of behaviour and the consequences which may follow if they are not adhered to. All the information should be available in languages other than English if required and should be clearly explained to those who cannot read. It is important that probation officers and social workers are aware of any difficulties offenders may experience (language barriers, hearing or reading difficulties) which may prevent them from fully understanding their obligations and relationship with the supervising officer. The exploration of these matters requires skill and sensitivity, as something which is taken for granted (for instance, that everyone should be able to read these days) may be far from the truth and such an assumption may cause severe embarrassment or guilt.

The national standards require that supervision is placed in the context of a 'supervision plan' which accounts for the timing, content, methods and outcomes of the sessions held between the parties (see Home Office et al., 1995:19-21). A copy of this plan, which should be formed in consultation with the offender, should be given to the offender within ten days of the making of the order. This plan is open to review and amendments as necessary in the course of supervision. A review should take place every three months to consider progress. It is a requirement that the offender attends a minimum of twelve appointments, normally weekly, with the supervising officer in the first three months of the making of the order. These can be reduced to six in the following three months; and thereafter meetings should take place at least once a month.

If offenders violate the requirements of their order, and if the failure is deemed not to be serious, they should be made to explain their behaviour within two working days. A record should be made of the failure to comply with requirements if the reason given is unacceptable and the offenders should be given a formal warning. Two formal warnings within any twelve-month period of the order may lead to 'breach proceedings'. However, if the failure to comply with requirements is deemed to be serious, proceedings under the

Criminal Justice Act 1991 can be taken at any stage in the order 'and without prior warning' (Home Office et al., 1995:22).

A *community service order* can only be imposed on anyone aged 16 years or over for an imprisonable offence. It can range between 40 and 240 hours. Its main objective is to 'punish' the offender 'by means of positive and demanding unpaid work' and to achieve 'reparation to the community'.

As in the case of the probation order, the first work session must start within ten days of the making of the order and relevant information including requirements and consequences that will follow if those requirements are not adhered to should be given to the offender. Once again, such information must take account of the offender's language, hearing, speech, reading or other difficulties and steps should be taken to ensure that such information is understood by the offender.

National standards stipulate that no more than 21 hours per week should be worked, that work should not conflict with the offender's entitlement to welfare benefits, and 'if unemployed, CS placements should not prevent the offender from being readily available to seek or take up employment' (Home Office et al., 1995:37). All hours of work done should be properly recorded but cancellations due to bad weather should not, unless the supervisor requires the offender to remain on site. In this case only up to half an hour can be credited for work performed (see Vass, 1984 for the background to these arrangements and the development of national standards). Half an hour can be credited for meal breaks, if taken in the course of work. In the past, travel time was also credited, at the discretion of supervising officers (Vass, 1984); under the national standards travel time to or from community service placements which exceeds half an hour should be credited but the overall total should not be more than 10 per cent of the hours prescribed.

As in the case of probation orders, offenders' behaviour must be monitored. Progress should be reviewed once a week and any apparent failure to comply with requirements should be acted upon within two working days. If the explanation is not deemed to be acceptable, the failure should be formally recorded as a clear instance of failure to comply with the order. In such cases, a formal written warning of the consequences should be given to the offender. 'At most two warnings within any 12 month period of the order may be given before breach proceedings are instituted' (Home Office et al., 1995:39). However, breach proceedings can be instituted at any stage in the order and without prior warning if the failure to comply is regarded as serious. If proceedings are contemplated, these should be initiated within ten working days of the offence committed.

The *combination order* combines probation with community service. The probation element must be for a minimum of twelve months and a maximum of three years, and the community service order of 40 to 100 hours. As in the case of community service, the combination order is available only for offences punishable with imprisonment.

The declared purpose of the combination order is to secure the rehabilitation of the offender; to protect the public from harm; and to prevent the offender from committing further offences (which are similar to the probation order's purpose). The other part reflects the basic tenets of the community service order: punishment and reparation to the community.

Supervision should commence within five working days and the first community service session is to take place within ten days of the making of the order. Information, requirements and expectations as well as reviews of progress, formal warnings and breach proceedings should follow the standards laid out with regard to probation orders and community service orders.

As in the case of the community service order, although the legislation stipulates (and expects) that combination orders are imposed on 'serious offenders', in practice this is not so. Courts appear to be over-zealous in imposing any sanction they regard as appropriate for the occasion if others are not seen to be appropriate. In 1993 out of nearly 9,000 combination orders made, 70 per cent were made in magistrates' courts and 7 per cent in the youth court for offences which could not be deemed to be 'serious' under the original intentions of the legislation (Criminal Justice Act 1991) and the national standards (Home Office et al., 1992). As a result the revised national standards (Home Office et al., 1995) 'recognise that the application of the combination order to a wider range of offenders is appropriate' (Home Office, 1995a:18).

The Crown Court or the youth court is empowered to make a *supervision order* for any offender aged 10 to 17 inclusive. An order may require the offender to be under the supervision of a probation officer or a social services department for a period of up to three years. Under the Children and Young Persons Act 1969 the court is empowered to make specific requirements that may be included in a supervision order. These are as follows: residence with a named person (section 12(1)); to comply with any directions given by the supervisor (section 12(2)); to participate in specified activities (section 12A(3)); to live in local authority accommodation for up to six months (section 12AA); treatment of a mental condition (section 12B(1)); to comply with education arrangements (section 12C); and to comply with such other provisions prescribed by the court (section

18(29)). Unlike the probation order, the offender is not required to consent to the making of a supervision order. Commission of a new offence while under an order does not normally render the offender liable to be sentenced for the original offence. If offenders do not comply with requirements and breach proceedings are initiated, they cannot be sentenced for the original offence; they may be fined or given an attendance centre order instead.

The purpose of the supervision order is not dissimilar to that of the probation order. An order's objective should be to secure the rehabilitation of the offender, to protect the public from harm, and to prevent the offender from committing further offences. Commencement requirements and standards, the supervision plan, record-keeping and review of progress, frequency of contact and procedure for the enforcement of an order, which apply to the probation order, also apply to the supervision order (see above, pp. 177–8). However, there are certain differences, particularly with regard to the involvement of adults in the process (for example parents or other carers). Under 'methods' the national standards for the supervision order stipulate 'working with others to resolve personal difficulties': this may include the offender's family, school careers office, local education authority, housing department, social security office, employment or training provider (Home Office et al., 1995:28). Reviewing progress should also involve the parents or other carers where appropriate. When enforcement of the order is required the parents of other carers should again be involved, and where formal warnings are given, the supervising officer should ensure that the offender and the parents 'or other responsible adult' understand the warning and its implications.

*Supervision before and after release from custody*
It is not just supervision of offenders sentenced to community penalties which practitioners need to be well informed about. There is also the work done with prisoners and supervision after release (see Williams, 1996). National standards cover

> the supervision by the probation service and local authority social services departments of offenders both before and after release from custody. The standard relates to those offenders sentenced to 12 months or more (excluding life sentence prisoners) and young offenders serving less than 12 months who are supervised under section 65 of the Criminal Justice Act 1991. It also applies to young offenders serving determinate sentences under section 53 of the Children and Young Persons Act 1993. (Home Office et al., 1995:43; for a discussion of what knowledge and skills are required, see Williams, 1996)

*Child protection*
Another area which requires attention is child protection in the context of working with offenders. Jones et al. (1992:139) put the case thus:

> The probation service is not of course primarily a child protection agency. However, there are two sets of circumstances in which probation officers can become involved with child protection issues:
>
> – When the service has an involvement with a member of a household where a child is considered to be at risk of physical, sexual, or emotional abuse or neglect;
> – When the service has an involvement with a client who is identified specifically as representing a risk to children.
>
> Between them, these categories embrace a range of possibilities including both statutory and voluntary clients, and those upon whom reports are being prepared.

As referred to in Chapter 4 in this volume, in such cases, irrespective of context, the welfare of the child is the first consideration and 'supersedes everything else' (Jones et al., 1992:139). As in other cases of good practice and the evidence that has accrued from the various inquiries into child abuse and neglect, the important thing is to know and follow procedures and guidelines laid down by official bodies or the employing organisation (for useful guidance see Jones et al., 1992: ch. 9).

*The effectiveness of intervention and sanctions*
Another aspect of knowledge which is essential in being a competent practitioner is familiarity with debates and research findings about the effectiveness of intervention, what methods appear to yield better results than others, what penal sanctions seem to promote more adjustment in the community and which seem to suit some offenders or types of offences more than others (see May and Vass, 1996, particularly chs 8, 10, 11 and 12).

Although the issue of effectiveness is far from clear and as a concept may imply different things to different people (see Vass, 1996), there is a body of knowledge which suggests types of intervention which may appear more positive than others. For example, according to Fischer (1976, 1978), supervision and counselling that follow a clear and structured approach to problems, enabling them to be discussed and understood by the participants, is more successful in achieving positive outcomes than work which lacks clarity, openness and concreteness. Similarly, probation effectiveness (rates of reconviction and diversion from custody) appears to increase when aims are clearly specified and pursued (Raynor, 1988).

Intensive supervision, which combines a clear structure with clear aims but is still processed via social work principles, appears to yield better results than had been anticipated (Mair et al., 1994). *In toto,* as Raynor (1996) suggests, there are three areas which provide a promising and fertile ground for delivering an effective service: good programmes are characterised by *targeting* offenders at high risk of re-offending and the circumstances which contribute to their offending; *content and delivery* are structured, with clear goals and means which are designed to maximise and reinforce learning; and effective programmes are guided by proper *management,* well trained staff who are concerned about effectiveness and adequate resources; finally, we will add, no programme can be judged, reviewed and amended for improvements unless it is *evaluated* (see Raynor and Vanstone, 1994).

There are, however, serious limitations to the above type of work. Although such structured and carefully planned work with offenders may yield encouraging results, it is expensive in the long term and as it is highly intensive, it is limited in its capacity to accommodate large numbers of offenders.

The evidence is not clear-cut about any form of intervention or penal sanction and the evidence may sometimes run contrary to expectation. For instance, it is not clear why offenders sentenced to a probation order with 4A/4B requirements (that is, with specific requirements) should have a higher reconviction rate (of nearly 10 per cent) than prison, 20 per cent more than straight probation and 14 per cent more than community service (Lloyd et al., 1994). However, one needs to be careful in interpreting such findings (Vass, 1996) because they may not mean that probation with day centre requirements is less effective than the rest. There are other factors which need to be taken into account (for example characteristics of offenders, the actions of supervising officers in reporting technical or real offences, the mechanics of law enforcement and so on).

This aspect of effectiveness is, as Raynor (1996) points out, neglected by national standards. Although national standards are designed to increase consistency and efficiency, they lack 'a primary focus on effectiveness'. For example, as Raynor adds, national standards do not differentiate between high- and low-risk offenders and yet there is evidence to suggest that supervision which may be appropriate for high-risk offenders may not be so for low-risk offenders.

In summary to this section on knowledge, the acquisition of 'intellectual qualities . . . [is] rooted in the very substance of working with offenders: a knowledge-base which serves to enlighten and critically evaluate the issues, contexts and outcomes of intervention' (Boswell, 1996) is a requirement.

## The essential skills of working with offenders

A skill is the ability to practise or perform tasks which demonstrate 'expertness'. A combination of knowledge, values and skills, we have argued, develops competence at expected standards. CCETSW (1995) specifies the areas where social workers and probation officers need to demonstrate competence. They need to be able to *communicate and engage, promote and enable, assess and plan, understand people and the impact of change, assess need and care planning, intervene and provide services, contribute to the work of the organisation, manage and evaluate their own capacity to develop professional competence.*

Chapter 3 covered the above, under the headings cognitive skills, administrative skills, interpersonal skills, decision-making skills and use and management of resources. These skills apply to every social context of work with offenders and it is not necessary to repeat them here. Nonetheless, when these different headings or concepts are looked at afresh (and in combination with knowledge and critical analysis) some specific skills become particularly evident as well as important in any situation which involves the supervision of offenders. As Boswell (1996) has provided a succinct summary of these essential skills, we will use her work to draw attention to their significant attributes. From Boswell's (1996) work, one can identify the following essential skills (see also Jones et al., 1992):

* communication (including listening, oral and written);
* assessment and evaluation (including report-writing and record-keeping (see Jones et al., 1992: ch. 10);
* intervention;
* relating knowledge to practice;
* forming and maintaining professional relationships;
* managing and coping with workload;
* use of self.

As the use of the self and self-awareness is a process which relates to every other skill at any given moment in time and social interaction, self-evaluation and critical self-appraisal becomes necessary. Boswell offers a framework for self-monitoring and self-evaluation as a basis for action which operates along normal 'research' lines. That is to say, in the same way in which one defines the topic, research topic, methodology, collection of facts, analysis and interpretations, conclusions and recommendations, a practitioner can also refer to a simple revision of that format by raising and acting on the following issues (Boswell, 1996):

1. What are my goals and desired standards?
2. What means are at my disposal to carry through these goals and what means exist for evaluating progress?
3. What knowledge do I have and how can it help me understand the issues, contexts and outcomes?
4. What are my own perspectives?
5. Collect and collate data (assessments, evaluations, record-keeping) which give you an indication of how you are doing.
6. Interpret the findings (which should answer the question 'what does all this mean?')
7. Use the findings to make recommendations (for example, 'how do I improve my performance?')
8. Review the performance at a later stage in the light of new developments and changes undertaken or imposed from outside.

**Conclusion**

In this chapter we have covered what we regard to be the most fundamental areas of knowledge, values and skills which combine with understanding to create competent practitioners. It is important to say that being 'competent' does not mean that there is a limit to what can be achieved: our argument has been throughout this book that nothing is static. Everything is changeable and negotiable. As such, what is competent in one instance and is transferable to another may require further changes and amendments to ensure that none of the components of that competence (knowledge, values and skills) remain isolated, static and dated. For proper and confident performance those constituent parts must work in synergy.

Having said that it must be stressed too that no individual should be regarded as 'incompetent'. As the Home Office Probation Training Unit (Probation Training Unit, 1994:1) recognises, 'We are all competent in different ways. We may think we can do some things well, but probably accept that there is always some room for improvement.' That is the gist of what good practice is: avoiding the urge to devalue others and ourselves but at the same time recognising that improvements are always called for.

CCETSW's own statement about competence in social work provides a useful summary with which to conclude this chapter (CCETSW, 1995:3):

Competence in social work is the product of knowledge, skills and values. In order to provide evidence that they have been achieved . . . students will have to demonstrate that they have: met practice requirements, integrated social work [probation] values; acquired and applied knowledge; and reflected upon and critically analysed their practice and transferred knowledge, skills and values in practice. . . . It is only practice which is founded on values, carried out in a skilled manner and informed by knowledge, critical analysis and reflection which is competent practice.

## References

Becker, H.S. (1963) *The Outsiders: Studies in the Sociology of Deviance*. London: Collier-Macmillan.

Blumer, H. (1969) *Symbolic Interactionism: Perspectives and Method*. Englewood Cliffs, NJ: Prentice-Hall.

Boswell, G.R. (1996) 'The essential skills of probation work', in T. May and A.A. Vass (eds), *Working with Offenders: Issues, Contexts and Outcomes*. London: Sage. pp. 31–50.

Bottoms, A.E. (1989) 'The place of the probation service in the criminal justice system', in Central Council of Probation Committees, *The Madingley Papers II* (mimeo). Cambridge: Institute of Criminology.

Bottoms, A.E. and Stelman, A. (1988) *Social Inquiry Reports*. Aldershot: Gower.

Broad, R. (1996) 'New partnerships in work with offenders and crime prevention work', in T. May and A.A. Vass (eds), *Working with Offenders: Issues, Contexts and Outcomes*. London: Sage. pp. 204–21

Buckley, K. (1996) 'Masculinity, the probation service and the causes of offending behaviour', in T. May and A.A. Vass (eds), *Working with Offenders: Issues, Contexts and Outcomes*. London: Sage. pp. 96–115.

Campbell, A. (1984) *The Girls in the Gang*. Oxford: Basil Blackwell.

Carlen, P. (1988) *Women, Crime and Poverty*. Milton Keynes: Open University Press.

CCETSW (1995) *DipSW: Rules and Requirements for the Diploma in Social Work*. (Paper 30), revised edn. London: Central Council for Education and Training in Social Work.

Cloward, R. and Ohlin, L. (1960) *Delinquency and Opportunity: A Theory of Delinquent Gangs*. Chicago: Free Press.

Cohen, A. (1955) *Delinquent Boys: The Culture of the Gang*. New York: Free Press.

Cohen, S. (1967) 'Mods, rockers and the rest: community reactions to juvenile delinquency', *Howard Journal of Criminal Justice*, 12: 121–30.

Cornwall, A. and Lindisfane, N. (eds) (1994) *Dislocating Masculinity: Comparative Perspectives*. London: Routledge.

Denney, D. (1996) 'Discrimination and anti-discrimination in probation', in T. May and A.A. Vass (eds), *Working with Offenders: Issues, Contexts and Outcomes*. London: Sage. pp. 51–75.

Dickinson, D. (1993) *Crime and Unemployment*. Cambridge: Department of Applied Economics, University of Cambridge.

Dobash, R.E. and Dobash, R.P. (1980) *Violence against Wives*. London: Open Books.

Downes, D. (1966) *The Delinquent Solution*. London: Routledge & Kegan Paul.

Downes, D. and Rock, P. (1988) *Understanding Deviance: A Guide to the Sociology of Crime and Rule Breaking*, 2nd edn. Oxford: Oxford University Press.

Durkheim, E. (1933) *The Division of Labour in Society*. Glencoe, IL: Free Press (original work, 1897).

Durkheim, E. (1970) *Suicide*. London: Routledge & Kegan Paul (original work, 1897).

Ellis, L. and Hoffman, H. (eds) (1990) *Crime in Biological, Social and Moral Contexts*. New York: Praeger.

Ericson, R.V. (1975) *Criminal Reactions: The Labelling Perspective*. Lexington, MA: Lexington Books.

Farrington, D.P., Gallagher, B., Morley, L., St Ledger, R.J. and West, D.J. (1986) 'Unemployment, school leaving and crime', *British Journal of Criminology* 26(4): 335–56.

Feldman, D. (1964) 'Psychoanalysis and crime', in B. Rosenberg, I. Gerver and F.W. Howton (eds) *Mass Society in Crisis*. London: Macmillan.

Field, S. (1990) *Trends in Crime and their Interpretation*. London: HMSO.

Fischer, J. (1976) *The Effectiveness of Social Casework*. Springfield: C.C. Thomas.

Fischer, J. (1978) *Effective Casework Practice*. New York: McGraw-Hill.

Geary, R. (1994) *Solving Problems in Criminal Law*. London: Cavendish Publishing.

Gelsthorpe, L. (1989) *Sexism and the Female Offender*. Aldershot: Gower.

Gelsthorpe, L. and Morris, A. (eds) (1990) *Feminist Perspectives in Criminology*. Milton Keynes: Open University Press.

Gilling, D. (1996) 'Crime prevention', in T. May and A.A. Vass (eds), *Working with Offenders: Issues, Contexts and Outcomes*. London: Sage. pp. 222–42.

Harris, R.J. (1980) 'A changing service: the case for separating "care" and "control" in probation practice', *British Journal of Social Work*, 10(2): 163–84.

Harris, R.J. (1988) 'The place of the probation service in the criminal justice system', in Central Council of Probation Committees, *The Madingley Papers 1988*. Cambridge: Cambridge Institute of Criminology.

Heidensohn, F. (1985) *Women and Crime*. London: Macmillan.

HM Inspectorate of Probation (1993) *Developing Efficiency and Effectiveness Inspections*. London: Home Office.

HM Inspectorate of Probation (1994) *Annual Report 1993–1994*. London: Home Office.

Hirschi, T. (1969) *Causes of Delinquency*. Berkeley: University of California Press.

Hirschi, T. (1979) 'Separate and unequal is better', *Journal of Research in Crime and Delinquency*, 16: 34–8.

Hirschi, T. (1986) 'On the compatibility of rational choice and social control recoveries of crime', in D.B. Cornish and R.V.G. Clarke (eds), *The Reasoning Criminal: Rational Choice Perspectives on Offending*. Berlin: Springer-Verlag.

Holdaway, S. (1996) 'The role of probation committees in policing the development of the probation service', in T. May and A.A. Vass (eds), *Working with Offenders: Issues, Contexts and Outcomes*. London: Sage. pp. 116–33.

Home Office (1992) *Gender and the Criminal Justice System*. London: Home Office.

Home Office (1995a) *Strengthening Punishment in the Community: A Consultation Paper*. London: HMSO.

Home Office (1995b) *The Probation Service: Three Year Plan for the Probation Service 1995–1998*. London: HMSO.

Home Office, Department of Health and Welsh Office (1992) *National Standards for the Supervision of Offenders in the Community*. London: Home Office.

Home Office, Department of Health and Welsh Office (1995) *National Standards for the Supervision of Offenders in the Community*. London: Home Office Probation Service Division.

Hood, R. (1993) *Race and Sentencing*. Oxford: Clarendon Press.

Hough, M. and Mayhew, P. (1985) *Taking Account of Crime: Findings from the Second British Survey* (Home Office Research Study no. 85). London: HMSO.

Hungerford-Welch, P. (1994) *Criminal Litigation & Sentencing*. London: Cavendish Publishing.

*Independent, The* (1995) 'Smoker on tube is jailed for beating doctor', 22 April.

Jefferson, T. and Walker, M.A. (1992) 'Ethnic minorities in the criminal justice system', *Criminal Law Review*, February: 83–95.

Jones, T., Maclean, B. and Young, J. (1986) *The Islington Crime Survey: Crime Victimisation ad Policing in Inner City London*. Aldershot: Gower.

Jones, A., Kroll, B., Pitts, J., Smith, P. and Weise, J.L. (1992) *The Probation Handbook*. Harlow: Longman.

Lemert, E.M. (1967) *Human Deviance, Social Problems and Social Control*. New Jersey: Prentice-Hall.

Lindesmith, A.R. and Strauss, A.L. (1968) *Social Psychology*, 3rd edn. New York: Holt, Rinehart & Winston.

Lloyd, C., Mair, G. and Hough, M. (1994) *Explaining Reconviction Rates: A Critical Analysis* (Home Office Research Study no. 136). London: HMSO.

Maguire, M. and Pointing, J. (eds) (1988) *Victims of Crime: A New Deal*. Milton Keynes: Open University Press.

Mair, G., Lloyd, C., Nee, C. and Sibbitt, R. (1994) *Intensive Probation in England and Wales: An Evaluation* (Home Office Research Study no. 133). London: HMSO.

Matthews, R. and Young, J. (eds) (1992) *Issues in Realist Criminology*. London: Sage.

Matza, D. (1964) *Delinquency and Drift*. New York: John Wiley.

Mawby, R.I. and Walklate, S. (1994) *Critical Victimology*. London: Sage.

May, T. and Vass, A.A. (eds) (1996) *Working with Offenders: Issues, Contexts and Outcomes*. London: Sage.

Merton, R.K. (1957) *Social Theory and Social Structure*, revised edn. New York: Free Press.

Messerschmidt, J.W. (1993) *Masculinities and Crime*. London: Rowman & Littlefield.

Nellis, M. (1996) 'Probation training: the links with social work', in T. May and A.A. Vass (eds), *Working with Offenders: Issues, Contexts and Outcomes*. London: Sage. pp. 7–30.

Pearson, G. (1983) *Hooligan: A History of Respectable Fears*. London: Macmillan.

Pearson, G., Treseder, J. and Yelloly, M. (eds) (1988) *Social Work and the Legacy of Freud: Psychoanalysis and its Uses*. London: Macmillan.

Pearson, G., Blagg, H., Smith, D., Sampson, A. and Stubbs, P. (1992) 'Crime, community and conflict: the multi-agency approach', in D. Downes (ed.), *Unravelling Criminal Justice*. Aldershot: Gower.

Plato, (1955) *The Republic*, trans. H.D.P. Lee. Harmondsworth: Penguin.

Plummer, K. (1975) *Sexual Stigma*. London: Routledge & Kegan Paul.

Probation Rules (1984) London: Home Office.

Probation Training Unit (1994) *Introducing Competences*. London: Home Office.

Quinney, R. (1970) *The Social Reality of Crime*. Boston: Little, Brown.

Quinney, R. (1974) *Critique of Legal Order: Crime Control in Capitalist Society*. Boston: Little, Brown.

Raynor, P. (1988) *Probation as an Alternative to Custody*. Aldershot: Avebury.

Raynor, P. (1996) 'Evaluating probation: the rehabilitation of effectiveness', in T. May and A.A. Vass (eds), *Working with Offenders: Issues, Contexts and Outcomes*. London: Sage. pp. 242–58.

Raynor, P. and Vanstone, M. (1994) 'Probation practice, effectiveness and the non-treatment paradigm', *British Journal of Social Work*, 24(4): 387–404.

Raynor, P., Smith, D. and Vanstone, M. (1994) *Effective Probation Practice*. Basingstoke: Macmillan.

Rock, P. (1973) *Deviant Behaviour*. London: Hutchinson.

Rose, A.M. (1962) *Human Behaviour and Social Process: An Interactionist Approach*. London: Routledge & Kegan Paul.

Ruggiero, V. and Vass, A.A. (1992) 'Heroin use and the formal economy: illicit drugs and licit economies in Italy', *British Journal of Criminology*, 32(3): 273–91.

Russell, D. (1982) *Rape in Marriage*. New York: Macmillan.

Schur, E.M. (1969) 'Reactions to deviance: a critical assessment', *American Journal of Sociology*, 75: 309.

Simon, R.J. (1975) *Women and Crime*. Lexington, MA: Lexington Books.

Smart, C. (1989) *Feminism and the Power of Law*. London: Routledge.

Smith, D. (1995) *Criminology for Social Work*. Basingstoke: Macmillan.

Smith, D. (1996) 'Pre-sentence reports', in T. May and A.A. Vass (eds), *Working with Offenders: Issues, Contexts and Outcomes*. London: Sage.

Sprack, J. (1995) *Emins on Criminal Procedure* 6th edn. London: Blackstone Press.

Stanko, E.A. (1987) 'Typical violence, normal precaution: men, women and interpersonal violence in England, Wales, Scotland and the USA', in J. Hanmer and M. Maynard (eds), *Women, Violence and Social Control*. London: Macmillan.

Stanko, E.A. (1988) 'Hidden violence against women', in M. Maguire and J. Pointing (eds), *Victims of Crime: A New Deal*. Milton Keynes: Open University Press.

Stone, G.P. and Farberman, H.A. (eds) (1971) *Social Psychology through Symbolic Interaction*. London: Ginn.

Sutherland E.H. and Cressey, D.R. (1966) *Principles of Criminology*. Philadelphia: T.P. Lippincott.

Taylor, I., Walton, P. and Young, J. (1973) *The New Criminology*. London: Routledge & Kegan Paul.

Taylor, I., Walton, P. and Young, J. (eds) (1975) *Critical Criminology*. London: Routledge & Kegan Paul.

Turk, A.T. (1969) *Criminality and Legal Order*, Chicago: Rand McNally.

Vass, A.A. (1984) *Sentenced to Labour: Close Encounters with a Prison Substitute*. St Ives: Venus Academica.

Vass, A.A. (1990) *Alternatives to Prison: Punishment, Custody and the Community*. London: Sage.

Vass, A.A. (1996) 'Community penalties: the politics of punishment', in T. May and A.A. Vass (eds), *Working with Offenders: Issues, Contexts and Outcomes*. London: Sage. pp. 157–84.

Walker, M.A. (1988) 'The court disposal of young males, by race, in London in 1983', *British Journal of Criminology*, 28: 441–60.

Walker, M.A. (1989) 'The court disposal and remands of white, Afro-Caribbean and Asian men (London, 1983)', *British Journal of Criminology*, 29: 353–67.

Ward, R. and Ward, S. (1993) *Community Sentences: Law & Practice*. London: Blackstone Press.

Wasik, M. (1993) *Emins on Sentencing*, 2nd edn. London: Blackstone Press.

Wasik, M. and Taylor, R.D. (1991) *Criminal Justice Act 1991*. London: Blackstone Press.

Williams, B. (1996) 'The transition from prison to community', in T. May and
A.A. Vass (eds), *Working with Offenders: Issues, Contexts and Outcomes*. London:
Sage. pp. 185–203.
Williams, K.S. (1994) *Textbook on Criminology*, 2nd edn. London: Blackstone
Press.
Wilson, J.Q. (1985) *Thinking about Crime*, 2nd edn. New York: Vintage Books.
Young, J. and Matthews, R. (1992) *Rethinking Criminology: The Realist Debate*.
London: Sage.

# 7

# Competence in Social Work
# and Probation Practice

In the previous chapters we covered the knowledge base, values and skills of social work. We then referred to three major social work areas of work (pathways): children and families; community care and social work with adults; and crime, probation and social work with offenders. In this final chapter we will cover the major competences which students and other practitioners (in any context of social work, including probation) need to demonstrate in practice for effective and reliable professional performance.

However, before we refer to practice learning and requirements for competent social work and probation practice, it would be useful to provide a brief summary of the major themes identified in the preceding chapters and how the three areas of knowledge, values and skills combine to create competent practitioners.

**Knowledge base**

We pointed out the need for practitioners to be rigorous in their acquisition of knowledge and be able to upgrade, improve, amend and select knowledge relevant to their practice. We argued that competence which is regarded as something acquired by merely learning a task (for example, as in the case of someone who is taught to follow procedure in fitting or repairing an electrical appliance) is not appropriate for social work and probation contexts. Merely learning a task without the ability to conceptualise and transfer information and ideas from one case or context of work to another (just because they are not identical or because they do not appear to share an affinity with each other) is insufficient. Such an approach leaves too many deficiencies, becomes an embarrassment, a hindrance to the task and effectively a serious liability.

For us, the above simplistic and mechanical approach to competence is not only unacceptable and inappropriate. We also consider it to be alien to the purpose of social work and probation practice. In our vocabulary, competence involves an intellectual ability which is based on a thorough coverage of all relevant information, arguments and facts which provide the cognitive tools for competent practice. For example, we would expect that a student of social and probation work would know about the place of social work and probation in this society; the role and tasks of practitioners and debates about care and control, authority and subordination; the diversity of personal, social, family and community structures and lifestyles; the components of effective communication with users who come from those diverse structures and lifestyles (which means knowing and understanding personal and social predicaments such as those of minority ethnic groups, young people, adults, offenders, people with physical or learning difficulties); inter-agency work and partnerships; statutory duties and powers, legislation relevant to children and families, community care and work with adults, criminal justice and mental health; theories and models of human behaviour and causes of crime; policy issues including penal sanctions and effectiveness; national standards for offenders, family court work and social work in general in the criminal justice system; working in and with groups (group work); principles and methods of assessment; community care legislation and models of contracting, purchasing and provision of services; research on effectiveness and its relevance to practice; the legal and policy context of work and the practice implications of social control, constraints and restrictions; issues about disengagement from working relationships and managing endings with service users; time management, resource provision and organisational theories; knowledge of self and use of self in social work and probation practice; sources and forms of oppression, disadvantage and discrimination based on race, gender, religion, language, age, class, disability and sexual orientation and their impact at the personal and structural level.

In other words, it is essential that 'students learn about and understand the legislative framework, philosophy and models of service delivery' (CCETSW, 1995:5), that they demonstrate core knowledge about the range of issues, methods and theoretical approaches relevant to social work and probation practice, and are able to make a critical analysis of that knowledge and selectively apply it in a skilled manner to their practice.

## Values

Knowledge on its own, without a moral framework, can lack both relevance and usefulness. Indeed it can also be dangerous, as it will know of no boundaries and its application will be another form of 'theology', a political form of correctness, which dismisses differences amongst individuals and groups, needs and methods amongst others and attempts to apply the same rules and perspectives to all people and circumstances. In that context, intervention or service delivery will be guided by a blind need to apply or impose the rules of conformity irrespective of circumstances. It is for that reason that social work and probation practitioners must adhere to a set of values which are clear but at the same time flexible enough to account for both the purpose of their work and the fact that the social context of that work is dictated by diversity.

The diversity is characterised by differences in religion, ethnicity, culture, language, social status, gender, sexual orientation, family structure, lifestyles and perceptions of 'normality' (for instance the way in which people with physical or learning difficulties, sensory or some other visual or perceived impairment are treated). It is expected that practitioners will be knowledgeable about such differences, be aware of their own values and prejudices and be reflective, and that they will base service provision on clearly assimilated values which guide their behaviour and interactions with users.

We have identified a number of core values throughout the book, whether in the context of working with children and families, or community care or offenders. Although each context of work may place more emphasis on some core values than others because of its peculiar characteristic of dealing with different user-groups, the same core values are, nonetheless, relevant to every organisational context of work. For instance, working with offenders requires particular emphasis on the values of respect for persons and care for persons. These, though they are core values for social workers in general, have a more specific meaning for probation officers because of the nature of their work. As probation officers are dealing, in the main, with a population of users who bear a serious and official stigma as a result of committing criminal acts against the law and the community and are subject to punishment, it is extremely easy to see them only in that capacity and treat them as alien people. In short, such values require to be at the forefront of work with offenders to remind practitioners that those individuals still need to be treated with dignity and respect; and, as we suggested in Chapter 6, to assist such practitioners to see as well as understand them as 'whole persons'.

In a sense, values are the foundation for the development of core knowledge and skills and their combined application to practice. The value base which we have referred to in this book accommodates a number of significant messages with regard to what service provision is, should be and ought to be. It should be guided by a belief (and translated into action) in the rights of the individual, the right to freedom from harm or abuse, the right to respect, the right to confidentiality, recognition of difference and diversity, a commitment to social justice (including recognition of supervision and control in the community as opposed to institutionalisation), and accountability (see also CCETSW, 1995:4).

## Skills

We argued that skills development is a bridge between exploring values, acquiring knowledge and translating these into positive service provision. A number of core skills, relevant to every social work context, were discussed and used to inform the different pathways covered.

In summary, we referred to the importance of developing analytic skills offering a capacity to conceptualise, critically evaluate and weigh up information and modes of intervention for the best choice and selection of appropriate and effective means of service provision. We argued that these cognitive skills must also incorporate research findings in practice and be flexible enough to apply to diverse contexts and user-groups. Interpersonal skills were also referred to which emphasise an understanding and awareness of the self in relation to others and how that interaction has social consequences for the participants. We emphasised the importance of establishing and sustaining working relationships with service users as well as agencies other than the practitioners' own, working with difference and diversity and negotiating conflicting demands (for instance, the interests of the child versus those of the family or the court, the interests of the offender versus the interests of the victim, the community, the court and political expediency). In addition, we stressed the importance of listening skills and communicating verbally, non-verbally and in writing (including via interviews and presenting reports to courts). Administrative skills (which include setting priorities, time management, managing workloads, keeping reliable records and using information technology) are important in social and probation work tasks. Record-keeping and report-writing are of particular significance to competent practice. The importance of recording information accurately and succinctly is paramount. Information should be completed and stored in accordance with statutory and legal requirements (if they apply) and with agency and inter-agency procedures.

Keeping records is an effective and practical way (when it is done carefully and efficiently) of reviewing progress, giving guidance, assisting service users to understand the purpose of supervision or their own actions and helping colleagues to be aware of work carried out with particular service users.

Most important of all, when reports need to be provided to courts (for instance in cases of breach of requirements of a community sentence) such records are essential in offering a clear history of events, and where necessary can be presented as evidence. In the HM Inspectorate of Probation (1994) report, serious shortcomings were uncovered in the recording of information. Similarly, the production of clear, precise and concise written communications including documents and reports to the courts (for instance pre-sentence reports) is absolutely critical in the creation of a competent service. Preparation of reports for courts (subject to national standards: see Home Office et al., 1995) was covered in some detail in Chapter 6 and it is an area which must be addressed by every social worker and probation officer. This is because such reports play a fundamental part in the quest for achieving the value of 'social justice'. Pre-sentence reports, for example, are documents which assist the courts to make or reach the correct decisions with regard to sentencing practices. If such reports are of limited relevance, badly written and prepared (for instance not following procedure, guidance and appropriate format specified in the national standards or are full of spelling errors) social workers and probation officers not only let themselves and their agency down, but also, and more importantly, service users. The HM Inspectorate of Probation (1994:30–31: paras 4.10–4.12) report identified serious deficiencies in this area and added that:

> A variety of practices was noted and disturbing differences in service ideologies were encountered. . . . The quality assessment of 214 PSRs revealed that 25 per cent were not of an acceptable standard. . . . 'Same day' PSRs scored lowest on the overall quality scores for the PSRs assessed (33 per cent were of an unacceptable standard). . . . Steps should be taken by all services to ensure that PSRs were of the required standard. . . . Above all, services should be more proactive in ensuring the provision of expedited reports, based on a nationally agreed and consistent policy.

The importance of presenting good reports to courts (criminal or civil) needs to be recognised by every service. One should expect all social workers and probation officers (working, say, in youth justice, criminal courts, and family work) to be skilled in the area.

Another skill which is of paramount importance for competent work is the ability to gather, record, evaluate and assess people's needs, rights, risks, strengths, responsibilities and resources. It is also important that an ability to evaluate the harm which may be caused by individuals' actions to others and ways of reducing that risk is present and properly demonstrated. In order to do this efficiently, practitioners must be able to devise a programme or a 'plan of intervention or supervision' which specifies the purpose of supervision, the goals, the means and the outcomes. As pointed out in Chapter 6, there is evidence to suggest that where such aims and means are clearly stated, reviewed and assessed together with service users there appear to be more positive outcomes than when work is done haphazardly and in an aimless, unchecked fashion.

It is essential to emphasise that the skill of making assessments and acting on them encompasses all types of social work, including working with offenders. In that instance, practitioners must also be able to assess the offence(s) and offending behaviour in the light of all the circumstances and at the same time evaluate and assess the risk to the public.

We also referred to the skill of contributing to the planning, monitoring and control of resources. Practitioners, we argued, should know about available resources, priorities, criteria and procedures for their deployment and ensure that resources are planned and used in efficient ways. It is a skill which in the past was deemed to be the prerogative of senior managers of a service whilst others were expected to remain oblivious or ignorant of budgeting and utilisation of resources. This was a distorted impression of what social workers and probation officers did but it succeeded in convincing the majority of practitioners that the best way to avoid thinking about it was to turn a blind eye to the availability, distribution and management of resources. This is no longer acceptable nor advisable. Social workers and probation officers have a duty to know about resource provision and priorities and must demonstrate skill in managing such resources in the best interests of their services and their users.

## Competence

Competence is a successful amalgamation of knowledge, values and skills together with a process of understanding one's own self and what effects that process has on others as well as on the outcome(s) of supervision, intervention and interpersonal relations with colleagues, users, and other agencies.

In sum, the argument we have put forward in a consistent manner is that the 'ability to perform, know and understand is called *competence*' (Probation Training Unit, 1994:1; emphasis in original). This ability, as the Probation Training Unit goes on to define it, means that a practitioner should be able to undertake a *variety of tasks* and activities at work and feel confident that the means and the outcomes of such activity will be the desirable goals. An able practitioner should be in a position to deal with a number of tasks and demands *at the same time*. That is to say, the tasks of social work and probation are such that more often than not the workload involves diverse and competing pressures and the practitioner should be in a position to utilise appropriate knowledge, values and skills to deal with this diversity as well as issues which happen or are referred to them at the same time. Although they can, and should, learn to prioritise their tasks and manage their workload, they cannot deny the fact that they are dealing with a variety of users of different ages and different backgrounds as well as different needs or requirements. They need to be able to set priorities but, like a competent juggler who can keep several objects in the air simultaneously, they must be skilled in negotiating and using appropriate means to handle different tasks and expectations which are happening simultaneously.

In view of that diversity and the 'juggling act', it follows that social work and probation practice are highly demanding in both mental and physical terms. Practitioners need to be constantly alert about their tasks and the way in which they respond to them. Since they are dealing with personal, interpersonal, criminal, moral and social issues and come across severe breakdowns in social relationships, they need to *manage pressure*, unpredictability, confusion, conflicting demands and unavoidable disruptions. The difficult task here is to remain competent without becoming overwhelmed by these demands to the point of reaching stalemate, loss of confidence and emotional saturation. They need to be capable of remaining involved and *meeting deadlines* (whether in writing reports or record-keeping, meetings or visits) whilst maintaining a distance from users' own lifestyles, needs and problem-presentations.

As we have suggested on a number of occasions a competent practitioner is not the one who manages (or wishes) to work alone, on an individual basis, but one who manages to establish workable and effective *links with other colleagues* within his or her own service or agency and with professionals who represent external agencies.

We have argued that social work knowledge, values and skills need to be seen as 'evolutionary'. They have a social career which is constantly expanded, defined, redefined and amended according to broader changes in the personal, social, political, moral and economic contexts. Competent practitioners, therefore, should adopt a similar position in their work. Social workers and probation officers should treat their holistic experience as a transactional exercise which is constantly in the process of 'becoming': perpetually developing and changing to remain relevant to the context and to prevent itself from becoming a sad and dangerous anachronism. In its broader sense, this dynamic experience requires social workers and probation officers to constantly question their knowledge, values and skills, amend them accordingly, and ensure that they are always congruent with new findings, ideas, theories, modes and methods of practice, expectations, requirements and procedures. It is only through such a competent approach that practitioners can claim they are efficient and effective and *accountable* to users, employers and the general public for their actions.

When all the above are put together, each practitioner must be able, when required, to offer evidence of conceptualisation, critical analysis, reflection and *transfer of knowledge skills and values* from one context of work to another. This professional competence must never be seen in static terms but as an ongoing process of learning, understanding and applying the necessary and most appropriate combinations of theory and practice for the most effective outcomes.

As a quick reference point for the reader, Figure 7.1 summarises the main components of knowledge, values and skills which combine to create competence.

### Practice competence

This section will offer a definition of different types of competence which arise from the above combination of knowledge, values and skills. This section will combine the major competences identified in this book and in social work and probation practice (CCETSW, 1995; Home Office, 1995a; Home Office et al., 1995; Evans, 1995; Pierce, 1995; Probation Training Unit, 1994) and present them in a schematic form. By indicating these competences and by identifying their major component parts and offering indicators of the type of activity which needs to be carried out for effective, efficient and reliable outcomes, students as well as practitioners can understand their work better and define the parameters against which their interventions and activities in the field take place. It is intended that these schematic presentations will be used as a quick reference point for students and practitioners and as a convenient means of monitoring standards and performance.

A good illustration of the effectiveness of such an approach to the promotion and development of competent practice is Middlesex University's *Professional Competence and Assessment Planner* (1994), developed by the School of Social Work and Health Sciences over a period of twenty-five years, which is now being used as a model of good practice by other social work and probation training departments in the country. The planner was the result of intensive and pioneering work by academic staff in collaboration with practice

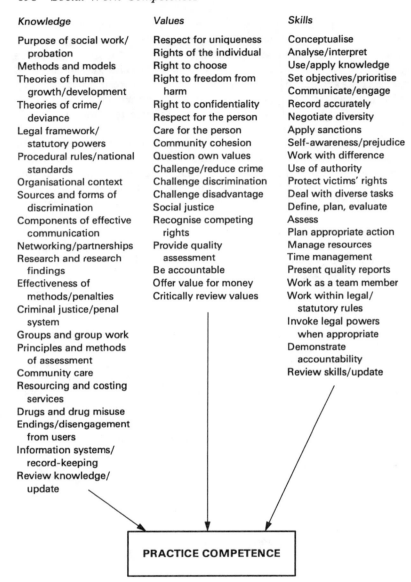

| Knowledge | Values | Skills |
|---|---|---|
| Purpose of social work/ probation | Respect for uniqueness | Conceptualise |
| Methods and models | Rights of the individual | Analyse/interpret |
| Theories of human growth/development | Right to choose | Use/apply knowledge |
| Theories of crime/ deviance | Right to freedom from harm | Set objectives/prioritise |
| Legal framework/ statutory powers | Right to confidentiality | Communicate/engage |
| Procedural rules/national standards | Respect for the person | Record accurately |
| Organisational context | Care for the person | Negotiate diversity |
| Sources and forms of discrimination | Community cohesion | Apply sanctions |
| Components of effective communication | Question own values | Self-awareness/prejudice |
| Networking/partnerships | Challenge/reduce crime | Work with difference |
| Research and research findings | Challenge discrimination | Use of authority |
| Effectiveness of methods/penalties | Challenge disadvantage | Protect victims' rights |
| Criminal justice/penal system | Social justice | Deal with diverse tasks |
| Groups and group work | Recognise competing rights | Define, plan, evaluate |
| Principles and methods of assessment | Provide quality assessment | Assess |
| Community care | Be accountable | Plan appropriate action |
| Resourcing and costing services | Offer value for money | Manage resources |
| Drugs and drug misuse | Critically review values | Time management |
| Endings/disengagement from users | | Present quality reports |
| Information systems/ record-keeping | | Work as a team member |
| Review knowledge/ update | | Work within legal/ statutory rules |
| | | Invoke legal powers when appropriate |
| | | Demonstrate accountability |
| | | Review skills/update |

PRACTICE COMPETENCE

Figure 7.1 *The making of practice competence*

teachers using as an example and base work done at North College of Advanced Education, Australia. Following the introduction of the Diploma in Social Work (CCETSW, 1991), the current Head of School redesigned the original document to meet new standards and requirements for the DipSW. Since 1992 (following those substantial amendments) the Programme Leader for Social Work Programmes has introduced relevant amendments on an annual basis to relate the planner to changes introduced by CCETSW, legal requirements, values or skills, thus maintaining the planner as a relevant learning tool in a fast-changing social, economic and political environment.

The same principle used in developing and presenting competences in the planner, albeit in less detail, is used here to make sense of the concept of competence. This is done by operationalising the main constituent parts of knowledge, values and skills discussed in this book. They are presented in the form of six major practice competences required by CCETSW (1995) in conjunction with specific requirements for probation officers articulated by the Home Office Training Unit, national standards, and other relevant material as applicable to social workers and probation officers. It is important that we make a few qualifications at the outset.

First, the presentation of the six competences and their operationalisation into components and indicators (that is to say, how they can be understood and identified in practice) does not mean that we have exhausted the full range of social work and probation work competences. Rather, we opted for those competences which are presented as requirements for good practice and whose application to practice not only leads to a successful completion of professional training but also confirms the standard of work required by the Diploma in Social Work (including probation training) for a professional career in social work.

Secondly, the operationalisation of these competences is not meant to imply that every social worker and probation officer needs to satisfy every aspect of those components or indicators. That is not possible. All we are offering is a heuristic device, an ideal situation in other words, against which competent practice can be understood, measured, and amended as appropriate. Indeed, as we said earlier, the list is not exhaustive and readers and practitioners can add more detail to those competences and can claim higher goals and achievements. It offers a foundation on which good practice can be constructed in a flexible and meaningful way. Indeed, no social work or probation student or practitioner will ever be in a position to meet *every* desirable competence with all its complex constituent parts. As CCETSW (1995:11) rightly points out, what is important is that practice 'must be sufficiently contrasting for students to gain a range of practice experience [and skills] and the opportunity to understand and demonstrate transferability of knowledge, values and skills, in practice'. It then goes on to add:

> In particular all students must demonstrate that they have met the practice requirements of Core Competence 'Assess and Plan', in work with service users who have significantly different needs and circumstances. . . . The evidence indicators for each of the practice requirements [competences], are provided as guidance to programme providers and students. The evidence indicators identify the activities that students would normally undertake, in order to gain evidence that they have met practice requirements. However discrete assessment documentation is not required for each evidence indicator, and the evidence that students will provide will vary in nature and emphasis, according to practice opportunities and the particular learning needs of students (CCETSW, 1995:11).

In short, what matters is not that every student and practitioner must satisfy every possible aspect of every competence (as that is impossible) but that they demonstrate quality, coherence and sufficient awareness and understanding of the issues and real life events they engage in. This point brings us to the third qualification. That although one can identify various competences which can be deemed of particular relevance to social work and probation practice, it is inappropriate to consider them as distinct entities. Such competences are interrelated and interlinked, and a competent professional is one who can demonstrate this interaction of the various constituent parts of different competences and put their common elements into practical effect. It is inappropriate for any student of social work and probation practice to remain oblivious to these connections and attempt to practise in a mechanical manner which excludes a view of the whole. We are back, therefore, to our previous argument that one cannot be competent without managing to offer a holistic approach (which incorporates knowledge, values and skills). We argued that competence is the product of a successful integration of these which is reflected in practice in the demonstration of the required standards of work. Similarly, as these are *competences* (as opposed to merely *a* competence) the same rule applies. These distinct competences are distinct only to the extent that they are defined and explained. In order to produce a consistently reliable and effective practice, they need to be integrated into a holistic approach for the achievement of specified tasks.

The final qualification that needs to be made is a reminder of our argument that social work and probation work are dynamic in their knowledge, values and skills. The same applies to competences.

There is always scope for improvement. Also, things change. Nothing remains the same over a period of time. Although the themes of this book, its major concerns, will remain the cornerstone of quality and will always be relevant and applicable to the evolving needs of the social work profession, the reader must constantly strive for improvements. These improvements cannot be achieved and attained without the practitioners constantly reviewing and updating their knowledge, values and skills. Competence cannot be improved further unless practitioners are willing to resort to their own efforts. They need to build on what is suggested in this book and regularly review their tasks and their outcomes in the light of new information that emerges as their practice goes through change and stages of development.

In the rest of the chapter we cover the core competences which accommodate both the official requirements and much of what has been referred to and discussed in this book. Each core competence is stated and subsequently analysed in terms of its core components and indicators.

*Core competence 1: communicate and engage*

*Components*

*Indicators*

Form, develop, sustain working relationships
— Take initiative in contacting/relating to colleagues within and outside the agency
— Consult with staff
— Communicate effectively
— Recognise differences/diverse perspectives
— Acknowledge shared values
— Understand roles/responsibilities/ statutory or other tasks of own organisation and other agencies
— Reconcile needs of offenders and communities
— Contribute to preventative work/ minimise risk
— Challenge attitudes and behaviour which lead to crime, cause distress, discrimination and harm to victims and others
— Maintain confidentiality

*Components*                          *Indicators*

Networking          ───────── Understand and communicate
                               effectively relevant matters including
                               resources
                             — Seek out, analyse and exchange
                               information
                             — Assess needs, offence, offending
                               behaviour and refer to or request
                               assistance from colleagues or other
                               agencies
                             — Accept and negotiate competing
                               perspectives and build on strengths
                               and expertise
                             — Encourage innovation, creativity and
                               flexibility in service provision

Service to the      ───────── Assess users' personal circumstances,
courts                         assist courts in reaching appropriate
                               decisions
                             — Present reports (including PSRs)
                               following guidelines and national
                               standards
                             — Supervise offenders given community
                               sentences
                             — Promote care for persons and their
                               families
                             — Respect persons and accept their
                               choices
                             — Offer assistance and supervision to
                               prisoners and their families through
                               direct work and through-care
                             — Apply constraints/controls as
                               required
                             — Invoke the law as required
                             — Promote practical support
                             — Recognise that individuals have
                               rights and responsibilities
                             — Keep accurate records
                             — Draw up supervision plans and set
                               objectives and means in conjunction
                               with users
                             — Know and understand relevant
                               legislation and apply as relevant.

*Components*                     *Indicators*

Self-awareness

- Identify, recognise own values/ prejudices
- Promote users' rights, privacy, confidentiality and protection
- Respect and value uniqueness and diversity
- Identify and combat discrimination
- Express hope for the future (believe in bringing out the best in people)
- Protect users and others from harm
- Challenge attitudes or behaviour (including offending) which leads to discrimination, harm, crime or fear of harm and crime

*Core competence 2: promote and enable*

*Components*                     *Indicators*

Promote rights of people at risk

- Balance needs of community and courts with those of users
- Assist users to represent their interests and rights
- Advocate on behalf of those who cannot do so for themselves
- Safeguard the welfare of children in family proceedings
- Assist offenders to lead law-abiding lives
- Supervise users in an open and constructive way

| *Components* | *Indicators* |
|---|---|
| Provide information and advice | — Facilitate access to information for users |
| | — Facilitate access to alternative services |
| | — Provide information as required by other agencies including courts, and respect confidentiality as appropriate |
| | — Seek out information and advice from others and update 'information bank' |
| | — Be known to others and use colleagues within and outside agency for advice |
| Assist users to improve their life chances | — Identify learning opportunities |
| | — Assist in reducing financial dependency through opportunities for education and training |
| | — Challenge a lifestyle which harms others (e.g. offending behaviour), carries penalties, severe stigma and reduces opportunities |
| | — Offer advice and assistance to users for dealing with emotional and practical difficulties |
| | — Challenge discrimination and treat all users fairly, openly and with respect |
| | — Earn the confidence of the public, courts and individual service users |
| | — Assist users to recognise their strengths, clarify goals, legitimise means and obstacles |

*Core competence 3: assess and plan*

| Components | Indicators |
|---|---|
| Assess and review needs/problems | Identify, evaluate context and purpose |
| | Collate and evaluate information |
| | Observe and assess behaviour |
| | Assess offence and offending behaviour |
| | Assess risk to the public |
| | Check (verify) information from various sources |
| | Record, store and maintain information |
| | Frame potential responses for recommendation, supervision, contact or diversion to other agencies |
| | Exchange information with staff and others |
| | Discuss and exchange information with users |
| | Produce, if required, clear, precise and understandable correspondence/documentation |
| | Produce, if required, clear, precise and understandable court reports |
| | Identify available resources and support networks |
| Identify, analyse risk of and to harm/abuse | Identify potential risk for users to harm others |
| | Identify potential risk for users to harm themselves |
| | Work in partnership with other colleagues/agencies |
| | Balance the users' and public's rights against assessment of harm |
| | Evaluate information/evidence for intervention following statutory requirements, procedure and national standards |
| | Demonstrate a working knowledge of the relevant legal and administrative procedures |

| *Components* | *Indicators* |
|---|---|
| Work according to statutory/legal guidelines | Know statutory, legal and administrative procedure and ensure application of national standards |
| | Explain to users their legal rights, the action to be taken within those legal boundaries and the implications if they fail to comply with requirements |
| | Ensure users understand the reasons for intervention |
| | Act according to those legal/statutory and national standards/rules |
| | Involve users at all stages of action and ensure that they understand the language/technical details |
| | Identify language barriers or other learning difficulties and use an interpreter |
| Negotiate and plan responses | Evaluate and apply research findings |
| | Consider options and reach choices |
| | Identify modes of intervention/action and justify |
| | Specify time scales for completion of tasks and for further reviews/action |
| | Involve users, carers and other professionals in identifying resources to meet agreed plans for action |
| | Identify and report any obstacles (including a shortfall in resources) which may retard progress and outcomes |
| | Produce and manage programmes for the supervision of offenders in the community |
| | Provide reports and advice to courts and others and represent agency in courts and other contexts |

*Components*

*Indicators*

Develop methods
of care, support,
protection
and control

- Cover work in accordance with statutory and legal requirements and national standards
- Manage and negotiate care and control
- Ensure users are clear about requirements and their role in the process
- Promote action in a manner which is likely to reduce distress to users and others
- Apply and enforce orders and licences where users fail to comply with court orders according to national standards
- Negotiate and confirm with users and other professionals and providers a combination of services
- Ensure clear messages are given to users about their tasks and obligations
- Clearly state who is accountable to whom

*Core competence 4: intervene/provide services*

| Components | Indicators |
|---|---|
| Develop action/ programmes of care, support, protection and control | Assist courts in reaching decisions about users |
| | Prepare and produce reports and other documents |
| | Use knowledge about methods of work, courts, partnerships, theories of causes of crime, penal sanctions, effectiveness, etc. |
| | Promote anti-discriminatory practice |
| | Work with all types of user, including prisoners and their families |
| | Address needs, offending behaviour and risk of re-offending |
| | Provide practical support |
| | Coordinate activity if it involves different services or other colleagues |
| | Monitor and evaluate the provision of care, support, supervision or control |

| Components | Indicators |
|---|---|
| Implement action | Select methods appropriate to the defined task(s) |
| | Negotiate and agree the aims, expectations and tasks according to clear rules for ongoing work |
| | Sustain and maintain working relationships |
| | Maintain a level of contact appropriate to the task |
| | Respond to expressions of emotional needs and offer support |
| | Agree time scales for work and reviews of progress |
| | Review changing circumstances and amend action plan(s) accordingly |
| | Understand and counteract discrimination; invoke legal powers if required |
| | Disengage from relationships at appropriate time and ensure users understand action |
| | Treat all users fairly, openly and with respect |
| | Respect users' choice but challenge behaviour which leads to harm to themselves and others |
| | Draw clear boundaries and expectations of behaviour |

*Core competence 5: working with organisation*

| Components | Indicators |
|---|---|

Assist in the improvement of service delivery

— Contribute to the planning, allocation and evaluation of work by groups, individuals and self
— Contribute to the planning, allocation and evaluation of the team's work
— Contribute to team and self-development and improve performance
— Set out clearly your role within the team
— Establish, maintain and enhance effective working relationships
— Establish and maintain reliability and trust
— Relate to authority and immediate supervisor
— Provide support to other colleagues
— Hold staff and self accountable for quality of work
— Enhance effective communication patterns between agency and service users
— Assess and evaluate team and self-performance

Assist to plan, monitor and control resources

— Assist in the planning and use of available resources
— Monitor and contribute to the control of resources
— Make suggestions for enhancing resource provision
— Devise plan for enhancing resource provision

| Components | Indicators |
|---|---|
| Evaluate effectiveness and efficiency | Seek feedback from colleagues and users |
| | Have defined criteria for measuring effectiveness |
| | Know available research findings |
| | Enable users to express their views on service received |
| | Discuss such expressed views with users, team and supervisors and respond accordingly |
| | Analyse the impact of self on those directly affected and their support networks |
| | Record evaluations and use to monitor future developments |
| | Share evaluations with team and learn from the experience |

*Core competence 6: develop professional competence*

| Components | Indicators |
|---|---|
| Use supervision effectively and manage workload | Use supervision in a constructive and informative manner |
| | Agree priorities and do not hesitate to explore professional matters in detail |
| | Act in accordance with expectations, role and responsibilities |
| | Develop coping techniques and ways of dealing with stress |

*Components*                          *Indicators*

Provide high-quality information, assessment and related services to courts/other users

- Provide accessible and timely pre-sentence reports
- Deliver national standards for family court welfare work
- Provide timely bail information reports
- Provide timely parole assessment reports focusing on assessment and management of risk to the public
- Develop measures to enhance the service's public profile and public understanding of the role of the probation service, social services or other agency in the welfare/criminal justice system

Maintain high standards of quality

- Offer provision for high-quality strategic planning
- Offer provision for financial planning, monitoring and control
- Assist in the effective deployment of self and other staff

Exchange, process and report information

- Participate in and contribute to staff meetings/discussions
- Provide reports/documents for colleagues and other professionals/agencies
- Provide reports to courts as necessary and subject to national standards
- Record, evaluate and store information according to agency guidelines, legal requirements, procedures and national standards

| *Components* | *Indicators* |
|---|---|
| Assist in the resolution of competing professional interests/conflicts | Acknowledge, identify and understand competing interests and possible conflicts |
| | Identify means of resolving difficulties/conflicts |
| | Negotiate differences and practise in an effective way |
| Reach decisions and make choices | Reflect on performance, tasks and challenges |
| | Clarify, verify and organise information necessary to decision-making |
| | Take responsibility for decisions and their outcome(s) |
| | Identify opportunities, circumstances, resources, etc. which could contribute to relevant decisions |
| | Identify obstacles to reaching decisions |
| | Identify means of overcoming obstacles |
| | Evaluate and discuss risks associated with decisions |
| | Record and store decisions with clearly stated rationale and means of achieving desired outcome(s) |

*Components* | *Indicators*

Critically evaluate and promote own professional development

— Welcome and contribute to appraisals and reviews of own knowledge, values, skills and practice

— Update knowledge, values and skills and integrate with new policies, legislative requirements, national standards, administrative procedure, research findings, etc.

— Integrate new knowledge, values and skills into practice

— Use agency staff development opportunities and assist in the enhancement of team performance

— Take responsibility for own continuing learning and development

— Remain, at all times, accountable for own professional competence

— Maintain, at all times, a sense of fairness and social justice

**Summary and conclusion**

In the last few years social work and probation work have undergone considerable change. Indeed, so much change that practitioners as well as educators are beginning to question their capacity to understand the rationale of such abrupt and continuous amendments to their working environment. CCETSW's introduction of a new set of requirements and a continuum of education and training in cooperation with major government, employer, educational and professional interests (CCETSW, 1991, 1995; Nellis, 1996) has had far-reaching effects on the quality, type and mode of education and training in social work. These effects are being felt in vocational qualifications in social care (NVQs and GNVQs); the professional studies and training for all social workers, including probation officers; practice learning for qualified social workers and probation officers who supervise DipSW students (for instance approval of social and probation work agencies as recognised practice settings and training and accreditation of practice teachers); post-qualifying education and training (in the form of a post-qualifying-level award and an advanced award); constant amendments to the requirements (hence a new and revised DipSW in the form of new regulations and expectations in regard to the competences relevant to effective social work and probation practice); new legislation (for example the Children Act 1989, National Health Service and Community Care Act 1990, Criminal Justice Act 1991, Criminal Justice and Public Order Act 1994, among others) and new indications from the government that more legislation is on the way to define or redefine the work of social workers and probation officers working in the criminal justice system (see Home Office, 1995b; Vass, 1996); and, perhaps far more relevant for the future of social work in this country, the revival and re-emergence of the old question of whether probation work is social work or whether it should be deemed to be a separate profession with its separate knowledge, values, skills and competences (Dews and Watts, 1994; Home Office, 1995c, 1995d; Nellis, 1996).

With so much change and transformation there is a real risk that social work and probation practice may lose their direction and what little credibility they have had with other agencies such as the courts and the public at large. This book has taken this threat seriously and has provided a detailed, critical and informative account of how practitioners can remain confident, efficient and effective through competent practice. The book is unique in its presentation of social work and probation practice. It has addressed conceptual and practice issues which others have taken for granted. It has unified knowledge, values and skills and applied them to particular pathways (children and families, community care and work with adults, crime, probation and work with offenders). And it has integrated the two parts to produce both an argument as well as a conceptual and practical tool (in the form of defined and operationalised competences) for use by students and practitioners.

As such we believe we have demonstrated that it is possible to bring together diverse and competing perspectives and practices and offer a unitary approach to the understanding, conceptualisation and practice of social work and probation.

Our integration of knowledge, values and skills with distinct (though interrelated) pathways to produce a set of competences which should be aimed at by students and practitioners has been guided and achieved by a strong belief that, irrespective of change and amendments to social work and the probation service which are imposed either by internal reorganisations of services or by outside political forces, the relevant themes and practices detailed here will always remain the main focus and core concerns of practitioners. The core knowledge, values and skills which inform practice and whose successful integration leads to competent practice; the interrelationship of pathways, albeit with their distinct focus subject to the characteristics of service users and relevant statutory, legal and administrative requirements; and the development of clearly stated competences which relate to efficiency and quality of performance in every social work and probation context form the gist of the subject-matter and practice orientation of social work and probation practice. Their relevance for the present and the future remains secured. We believe that students and practitioners of social work and those working with offenders will find this book of particular assistance in understanding, learning, appreciating and negotiating core requirements in their quest for competent practice.

In conclusion, we need to emphasise the fact that competent practice requires an integration of knowledge, values and skills and a constant search for learning and development. It is folly to consider that social work and probation skills can be learned and practised merely by rehearsing past events. It is important that practitioners learn to be self-critical and to aim at promoting their efficiency and effectiveness by continuous education and training. Without this, practice becomes dated and in many respects a risky business. For example, if it is necessary to resort to knowledge with a legal basis when working with children and families, community care and adults, or offenders, and the practitioner is using legislation which has been superseded by other laws, his or her practice will be marred by incompetence and serious failures in regard to outcomes.

We now come to the most difficult aspect of social work and probation practice (a point raised elsewhere: Vass, 1987). Social work in general is a social relationship. Whether it is probation with offenders or work with adults or children, the common denominator is that such work is done with people, for people and by people. By their very social nature, social workers and probation officers will always have to wrestle with competing perspectives, contradictory and ambivalent expectations of their tasks and functions, and will always be in the middle of conflicting social, political, ethical and moral imperatives. As their actions are determined by the social contexts within which social relationships develop or break down, their actions and decisions will always carry a social and moral risk: decisions which may be deemed rational and professional in one context – and provide the precedent for other similar situations – may be deemed (if new changes in legislation, requirements, guidelines, procedures, attitudes and expectations are not taken into account) irrational and incompetent in another. This is an inherent risk in social work as well as probation. Social workers or probation officers, irrespective of how competent and informed they are, must accept that they will always be standing at the moral crossroads of personal, organisational and societal cultures and responsibilities.

They will not, and should not, be (as that can prove disastrous in practice), genuinely confident or 'absolutely' efficient when confronted with service users, or a social problem, say child abuse and neglect, or crime and offenders, or when having to diagnose cause and effect or prescribe appropriate action. Uncertainty is the gist of social work and probation practice. Social workers and probation officers exist and perform in the grey areas of social life where exact solutions and measurements cannot be possible. Indeed they should not pretend, or be expected to pretend, by inflated claims about competences that they can find exact solutions or that their fortunes will improve by resort to new methods of vocational training (such as NVQs and GNVQs). The danger is that such vocational training may in fact destabilise the synergy which exists between knowledge, values and skills and the emergence of competences may neglect and impair the intellectual development of practitioners. Their capacity for analytical and informed practice will be severely curtailed and undermined.

Social workers and probation officers, therefore, must always accept those social risks and *act cautiously*. Every case they deal with and every social issue or problem that confronts them is unique. So whilst it is possible to generalise and show students and practitioners what to do in certain circumstances an open mind is essential and each case must be considered a 'special' case, in order to reduce or minimise risk. That is also why it is imperative that an amalgamation and integration of knowledge, values and skills take place for effective practice. For such a combined effort, together with a constant eye on advice and administrative procedure laid out by statutory and agency rules (for instance in cases of child protection and neglect), helps to ensure that those inherent risks are kept at bay.

Practitioners must maintain that synergy and promote good practice if they wish to be recognised and valued for what they do. At the same time there is a clear message for social work and probation practitioners: that social work (including probation) is not just a science. Maybe it is not a science at all, in the usual definition of the concept, though that is another matter. Rather, it is a form of 'art' (England, 1986). As with any piece of art, it is not the quantity which emphasises its value. It is the message, the insights and the meaning that are generated and interpreted by others which give any art its priceless value. Social workers and probation officers should take more notice of their art and should be encouraged to evaluate their own work and consider it as an important and effective way of keeping society together and assisting in the quest for social justice. They have a role, and an important one at that, to play in the social structure. Finally they should recognise their own art as something which is valuable and worth preserving for future generations of social workers and probation officers and for service users who will continue to benefit from them. But to achieve that, and to ensure that others interpret them in the same light, they should remember to practise the art of effectiveness which if paraphrased goes something like this: 'it ain't what you do, it's the way you do it, that's what counts!' It is not *what* social workers and probation officers do that matters but *how* they do it. This book has given much consideration to the 'hows' of the tasks and how practitioners can develop into efficient professionals. It is worth waiting to see if the message has been successfully transmitted and received. Time will tell.

## References

CCETSW (1991) *DipSW: Rules and Requirements for the Diploma in Social Work* (Paper 30) 2nd edn. London: Central Council for Education and Training in Social Work.

CCETSW (1995) *DipSW: Rules and Requirements for the Diploma in Social Work* (Paper 30) revised edn. London: Central Council for Education and Training in Social Work.

Dews, V. and Watts, J. (1994) *Review of Probation Officer Recruitment and Qualifying Training*. London: Home Office.

England, H. (1986) *Social Work as an Art*. London: Allen & Unwin.

Evans, R. (1995) 'CCETSW revised paper 30 requirements and probation officer core competences', letter to Rachael Pierce, Assistant Director, Education and Training, CCETSW. London: Home Office Training Unit, 20 March (mimeo).

HM Inspectorate of Probation (1994) *Annual Report 1993–1994*. London: Home Office.

Home Office (1995a) *The Probation Service: Three Year Plan for the Probation Service 1995–1998*. London: Home Office.

Home Office (1995b) *Strengthening Punishment in the Community: A Consultation Paper*. London: HMSO.

Home Office (1995c) *Review of Probation Officer Recruitment and Qualifying Training. Discussion Paper*. London: Home Office (mimeo).

Home Office (1995d) *Review of Probation Officer Recruitment and Qualifying Training. Decision Paper by the Home Office*. London: Home Office.

Home Office, Department of Health and Welsh Office (1995) *National Standards for the Supervision of Offenders in the Community*. London: Home Office Probation Service Division.

Middlesex University (1994) *Professional Competence and Assessment Planner*. Enfield, London: School of Social Work and Health Sciences, Middlesex University.

Nellis, M. (1996) 'Probation training: the links with social work', in T. May and A.A. Vass (eds), *Working with Offenders: Issues, Contexts and Outcomes*. London: Sage. pp. 7–30.

Pierce, R. (1995) 'Response to Rick Evans, Head of the Home Office Training Unit' (internal communication). London: Central Council for Education and Training in Social Work, March (mimeo).

Probation Training Unit (1994) *Introducing Competences: A Guide to Probation Service Staff*. London: Home Office.

Vass, A.A. (1987) 'CCETSW's prescriptions for change', *Social Work Today*, 18(20): 27.

Vass, A.A. (1996) 'Community penalties: the politics of punishment', in T. May and A.A. Vass (eds) *Working with Offenders: Issues, Contexts and Outcomes*. London: Sage. pp. 157–84.

# Index